IF NOT NOW, WHEN?

CHAIR YOGA

12-MINUTE PRACTICE TO STRENGTHEN BONE HEALTH

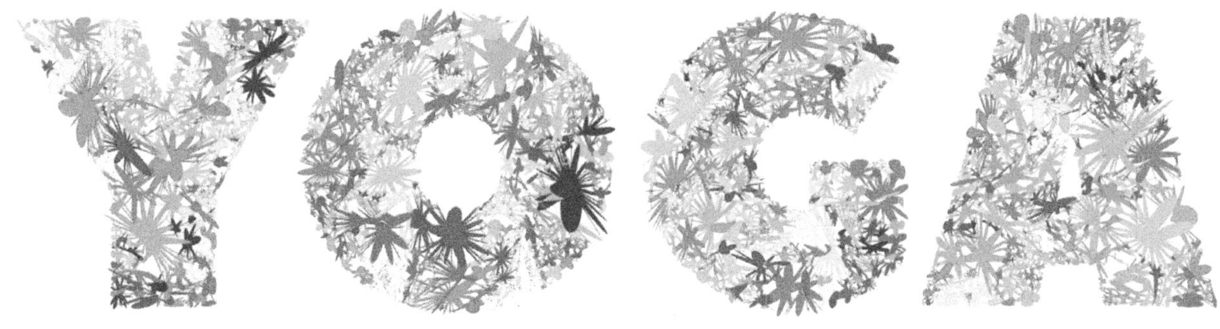

LARGE PRINT

MAKE THE MOVEMENTS SAFE AND ENJOYABLE FOR ALL BODIES TO LOSE WEIGHT, RECOVER ENERGY, CONCENTRATION AND RELEASE TENSIONS

STEP BY STEP FULLY ILLUSTRATED

Rebuilding Your Body

FLEX CLASS

FLEX CLASS

is an independent publisher, if you enjoy this book, please consider supporting us by leaving a review!

Unlock the Taste of Wellness!

Scan the QR code below to access an exclusive selection of **QUICK AND HEALTHY RECIPES**, perfectly complementing your journey with Chair Yoga.

Enjoy enhancing your wellness journey
with flavors that nourish your body and soul.

We want our books to be truly enjoyable for everyone.

TABLE OF CONTENTS

INTRODUCTION

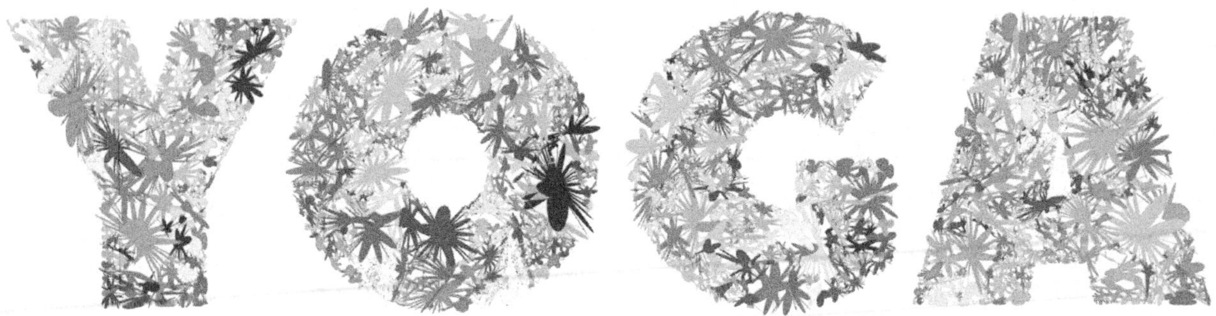

If thinking about yoga reminds you of long-limbed, flexible bodies in contortionist positions, try thinking again. Modern yoga has had an incredible development compared to yoga a thousand years ago, even just years ago.

Yoga has come to involve everyone and benefit everybody, age and mobility.

An example is given by **CHAIR YOGA**, THE YOGA THAT IS GOOD FOR EVERYONE. In this book we see together who it is for, where it can be practiced, the benefits and much more.

Chair yoga was originally intended for people with reduced mobility, whether due to trauma, illness, or age. Over the years, however, it has also become an essential tool for those who work in an office and spend many hours sitting, for those who travel a lot by plane and for pregnant women and for those with weight problems.

Just as the yoga positions on the mat increase flexibility, strengthen muscles, relieve pain, cramps and fatigue and calm the mind, in the same way the asanas practiced on the chair help body and mind bringing numerous benefits and advantages.

WHO IS CHAIR YOGA FOR?

- Elderly people
- Pregnant women
- Those with reduced mobility
- People in wheelchairs
- Sedentary workers
- Those who travel a lot, by train, plane or car
- People who have suffered physical trauma and are recovering
- Overweight people
- People with degenerative diseases
- Beginners
- People with balance problems

REALLY ANYONE WHO WANTS TO START YOGA IN A GENTLE WAY

Chair Yoga is aimed at everyone, even the most advanced practitioners. Who hasn't found themselves having to sit for hours? Chair yoga is a great ally to relieve the tensions that this position can build up on the back, hips and shoulders.

WHERE YOU CAN PRACTICE?

- At the office
- In the train, plane, car
- In a specialized yoga studio
- In a specialized physiotherapy center
- In the kitchen, living room, bedroom
- On holiday

WHEREVER YOU HAVE A CHAIR AVAILABLE

Chair Yoga, just as the name implies, is a yoga style that includes asanas, meditation and pranayama, practiced while sitting. For this reason, its practicality is enormous and it has infinite possibilities. Maybe someone in the office will look at you wrong, but seeing how your face relaxes by relieving muscle tension, they will want to try it and experience it too.

CHAIR YOGA, THE MAIN ADVANTAGES

We know the advantages and benefits of yoga well. Here, we add that also chairyoga brings infinite ones precisely because it is designed for those who need it most, thanks to the comfort of a stable and common position like that of a chair.

Scientific studies show the physical and psychological benefits of yoga. Incorporating it into your weekly routine helps improve health, noticing the difference from the very first lessons with a feeling of relaxation and comfort inthe body. Practice decreases muscle tension and joints become more mobile andfreer so that even basic activities, such as tying your shoes, become more feasible. And you can lose weight, as with traditional yoga.

In the practice of Chair Yoga most of the asanas can be performed with a chairmaking them possible for every body type, flexibility, mobility and level.

THE PHYSICAL BENEFITS:

STRENGTHENS THE MUSCLES. With advancing age, muscle tone tends to lose mass, increasing the risk of trauma. An accident, fall or any other trauma requires adequate recovery time. The different postures that can be practiced on a chair help to tone the body, (re) building a muscular structure able to support it better during daily activities.

IMPROVES POSTURE. For people with weight problems this yoga is great for improving the posture of the whole body. The positions to be maintained helps and strengthens the back muscles of the body without neglecting the abdominalpart.

CONTROLS YOUR WEIGHT. For many overweight people, starting physical activitycan be a big problem, because of the risks that being overweight entail and because of the volume of the body. Chair yoga is an alternative to fitness. Increasing muscle mass helps increase metabolism, rebalancing the general functioning of all organs and making them work better by contributing to keep weight under control.

INCREASES FLEXIBILITY. Older people or people with reduced mobility have excellent results from exercise by improving and increasing the range of motionof the whole body.

HELPS REDUCE PAIN. Practicing yoga two or three times a week helps to strengthen the muscles and oil the joints, making them stronger and consequently decreasing pain.

IMPROVES BODY CONSCIOUSNESS. Proprioception allows us to understand the movement of the body in space and to coordinate the movements accordingly. Especially for older people it decreases, increasing the risk of falls and injuries.Chair yoga helps you have better control of your body and movements leading tobetter movement.

THE PSYCHOLOGICAL BENEFITS:

KEEPS THE MIND ACTIVE. For people with degenerative diseases, Alzheimer's patients and elderly people, keeping the mind as well as the body active is essential for better functioning of the whole organism. Keeping the mind activehelps keep the spirit alive and healthy.

REDUCES STRESS AND ANXIETY. This is especially true after disease or trauma. One of the greatest benefits of yoga is to have a positive effect not only on the body but also on the mind, thus also improving the quality of life.

IMPROVES THE QUALITY OF LIFE. Yoga as a therapy is for any type of trauma. Chair Yoga improves the body structure of the individual both externally with flexibility and strength and internally with relaxation and calm. In this way, thosewho practice it benefit from it at every level.

Other benefits:

EASY TO PRACTICE. All it takes is a chair and your body. Great for taking a breakfrom your computer, at the office, at home or while traveling.

Finally, remember that **CHAIR YOGA** is a good introduction to the benefits of yoga practice, to stay active while decreasing stress, anxiety, pain and the consequences of illness or trauma. Improving the state of one's body improves the state of mind and consequently also the quality of one's life.

Are you ready to grab a chair and get started?

WHY DOES YOGA HELP YOU LOSE WEIGHT?

Today the practice of yoga is widespread all over the world, but have you ever wondered what its origins are?

Surely you will all know that it has its roots in the East, but there are many interesting things to know if you are approaching this discipline that involves theperson entirely: BODY, MIND AND SPIRIT.

The benefits that can be drawn from the practice of yoga are many, for both the body and the mind, and among these there is weight loss, if also accompanied by a healthy and balanced diet. By combining these two aspects, yoga will help you tone and make your body more elastic at any age! Two characteristics are enough: willpower and a lot of patience, in line with Zen philosophy!

ORIGINS AND CHARACTERISTICS OF YOGA

The Sanskrit term "yoga" indicates meditative and ascetic practices and many scholars identify a correlation between the term itself and the root "yuj-" whichmeans "to unite". Hence the meaning of the word yoga as a union of all parts ofthe person, therefore body, mind and spirit, and as a government of the senses by the conscience to obtain a perfect balance.

ONE OF THE FIRST testimonies that indicate the knowledge of meditation practices and mental and body self-control dates back to the third millennium BC, in the Indus River valley, in today's Pakistan, and it is a seal that depicts a human figuresurrounded by animals, sitting in a yoga position.

This testimony, therefore, dates back to well before the Arians settled in India.This population settled between 1500 and 1250 BC. in Punjab and wrote books, the "Vedas", which contain all their beliefs and philosophy, including referencesto yoga. Within these books there are no references to yoga as a real discipline,but there are various concepts related to this discipline. In the "Upanishads", thelast part of the Vedas, written between 800 and 300 BC, there are also referencesto practices with their effects.

THE "YOG-SUTRA" is considered to be the most authoritative ancient text which has yoga as its subject. Its author, the philosopher Patanjali, lived in the secondcentury BC. and he wrote this text which is made up of 139 aphorisms, the sutras,with which he expressed, in a very hermetic and concise way, concepts and ideas. The dating of the work is very uncertain but with it, yoga became part ofthe six philosophical systems of ancient India: the darshanas. This term properlyindicates "vision" and alludes to the conception of reality that derives from the practice of an ascetic and contemplative discipline.

Today the term yoga identifies a set of practices that also integrate other philosophies, developing many types of yoga, such as Buddhist, Tibetan Taoist and so on, and also differentiating according to style, for example the Ashtanga style, the Kundalini style and Hatha style.

In particular, the most popular yoga practices for weight loss at the moment areHatha and Vinyasa, but pay attention - there are differences!

HATHA YOGA CLASSES focus on the importance of muscle and postural lengthening and the importance of breathing. Its goal is to create a space between musculartensions, configuring itself as a gentle but not too gentle practice. By modulating movement and breathing, we also work on the attenuation of physical and mental stress. In practice, postures, sun salutation, meditation and relaxation techniques follow one another.

VINYASA YOGA, on the other hand, is much more dynamic, strong and fast, wherethe physical movement is synchronized with the breath. Its goals are to work onflexibility, strengthening muscle tone and making the transition from oneposition to another fluid.

Unlike other sports, YOGA DEVELOPS ALL PARTS OF THE BODY. This is because the combination of the different positions allows you to work all the muscles of thebody, also obtaining benefits for the nervous system. Yoga (but actually constantexercise) has been proven to make the body more flexible, improve posture andspeed up metabolism when combined with balanced and healthy eating habits.

Everyone can practice it and at any age. The only trick is to startwith lessons with a level for beginners, in order to gradually get in touch with your body without stressing it.

The combination of positions (asanas), meditation and breathingcontrol (pranayama) are able to bring not only benefits to the body but also to the mind, obviously if yoga is practiced consistently.

As for the positions, each movement involves a gentle and slow stretching of the muscle, which also acts on circulation and elasticity, preventing or mitigating pain due to muscle stiffness. The asanas therefore tone the muscles and also improve the perception of one's body, as well as massaging the internal organs.

Meditation is a very deep relaxation method that has the sole purpose of freeingone's mind from stress, anxiety or any other tension, thus giving a sense of well-being.

BREATHING CONTROL, on the other hand, helps to increase concentration and, in addition to providing the right amount of oxygen to the muscles, allows you to easily eliminate lactic acid and lower your heart rate.

PRACTICING YOGA can affect bowel movements and, therefore, can help resolve constipation or indigestion problems and a swollen belly. It strengthens the joints, tones the body, makes the spine more elastic, reduces muscle pain and improves elasticity, as it relaxes the muscles and connective tissues.

As already mentioned, practicing yoga helps CONCENTRATION AND CHANNEL ENERGY touse it in a positive way. It reduces stress and anxiety and strengthens self-esteem. In fact, meditation allows you to have positive thoughts and consequently helps you to better manage the daily situations of your life.

Another very important benefit of yoga is to help you ACHIEVE A HEALTHY WEIGHT. Practicing yoga to lose weight certainly provides greater self-awareness and helps to understand your body, also helping to distinguish true hunger from feeling hungry. Furthermore, as we have seen, yoga involves the whole body andaids digestion.

BUT IS YOGA CERTAIN TO HELP YOU LOSE WEIGHT? A study conducted by the Fred Hutchinson Cancer Research Center in Seattle found a correlation between the practice of yoga and weight loss: on a sample of 15,000 healthy middle-aged adults, both women and men, people who regularly practiced yoga, that is 30 minutes at least once a week for 4 or more years, they put on 3 kilos less in 10 years than the others who did not practice it.

The most interesting thing is that overweight people who had practiced yoga hadlost an average of 2 kilos, while those who had not practiced it had gained an average of 6 kilos in 10 years.

According to the researchers, this result was not linked to the calories consumedthrough yoga, given that few people practice aerobic yoga such as to make them lose weight, but it was linked to the effect on the mind derived from the practiceof yoga: a greater awareness of one's body allows you to perceive one's sense ofsatiety and makes it easier not to give in to temptations and to respect one's limits before overcoming them.

There are a lot of yoga poses and all of them are beneficial to the body. Someof these can help you reach your goal of losing excess weight. Remember that excessive gymnastics and sudden weight loss will not make you burn fat or firm the abdominal part, but only the commitment to combine healthy lifestyles thatare calibrated to your energy.

The best way to carry out a correct sequence of movement or positions is to follow some specialized instructor, but in the course of the book we will give yousome tips to do yoga exercises even in a home version but always in safety.

Have you ever thought that doing yoga at home could be one ofthe most effective methods for keeping yourself healthy and, atthe same time, for ensuring eternal beauty?

Practicing yoga can also help you lose weight as long as it is combined with a healthy and balanced diet, choosing fresh ingredients and superfoods. Try to enrich your daily diet with recipes such as puffed quinoa shots with nuts, blueberries and yogurt, and an avocado smoothie to boost your day, or quinoa and pumpkin meatballs and purple soup for lunch or dinner. The body will needto get used to it gradually, so it is good to avoid drastic diets to speed up the time: the secret is consistency and a lot of willpower.

Remember that BREATHING IS VERY IMPORTANT in all asanas and, depending on the exercise, one breath will be suitable instead of another.

The general rule is to create a routine that includes physical activity and healthy nutrition, making it a real lifestyle.

THE BENEFITS OF YOGA

You're interested in the world of yoga, but think it's out of your league because you are overweight. Wrong! Yoga for those who are overweight helps burn fat and control anxiety.

There are many public figures who practice yoga and confirm its health benefits. Indian Prime Minister Narendra Modi has proposed making this discipline a matterof national concern, so that everyone can benefit from it in daily life.

The Indian minister has even published a series of videos in which he himself, inan animated version, performs various yoga positions. In them he ensures us thatit is a healthy choice for everyone.

Do you need other reasons to prove the usefulness of yoga forthose who are overweight? We'll give you at least ten.

YOGA FOR THOSE WHO ARE OVERWEIGHT: THIS IS WHY IT'S USEFUL

1. **Improve your breathing**

   Yoga helps you breathe better and more consciously. With exercise and healthyeating, you will be able to burn fat much more easily.

   Being more aware of breathing and leading a more peaceful life allows nutrientsto reach the organs in the best way.

2. **Increase confidence and self -esteem**

   Yoga for overweight people is a great way to start leading a more active lifestyle.It is ideal for people who suffer from low self-esteem and insecurity.

   The progress made, on the physical and spiritual level, renews the perception ofoneself and the way in which life is approached. You will have more control overthe body: physical activity can really improve our life.

3. **Fight depression**

   Overweight people can, as we have said, suffer from low self- esteem, a risk factor for depression. This is the result of the insecurity they feel about their own body and appearance.

Doing yoga can help treat mild forms of depression. In addition, it is a discipline that leads to reflection, meditation, gaining confidence and maintaining an active life.

4. **Relieve Stress**

   The breathing and meditation exercises, applied to the positions during the yogaclass, help relieve stress and relax. You will be more focused on mental and physical work and more determined.

   Taking a moment of the day for meditation and deep breathing significantly reduces the levels of cortisol, the stress hormone. Getting used to filling your lungs with air will allow you to become more calm, useful in decisions and to face daily challenges.

5. **Reduce physical discomfort**

   Yoga for those who are overweight is a useful exercise to calm headaches, lowerblood pressure, fatigue and insomnia. These effects are due to an increase in oxygenation of the brain and the disposal of toxins, as a result of deep and harmonious breathing.

   As you progress, you will feel more encouraged to take other actions that help you lose weight. You will feel more energy and motivation towards healthy foodand good habits.

6. **You will notice progressive changes**

   No matter what your waist measurements are, in no case are they an impedimentto yoga practice. The important thing is not to ask the body for more than it cangive. You will be able to take on even the most difficult positions as you gain flexibility and confidence.

   The gradual effort required is ideal because it allows you to get used to it and never feel discouraged.

7. **It is a low impact activity**

   Yoga is a good ingredient for a healthy lifestyle that does not require drastic changes.

8. **It has positive effects on the endocrine system**

Each yoga position acts on a part of the body, on a muscular, nervous and hormonal level. Some of them are particularly indicated in case of thyroid disorders.

9. Fight anxiety

We have already mentioned the spiritual benefits and relaxing power of yoga, which is why it is considered an activity capable of reducing anxiety levels. This is thanks to the meditation and deep breathing required by the discipline.

The effects of yoga on the nervous system increase the desire to take care of one's body, as well as reduce the constant desire to eat. It will therefore affect the choice of a correct diet.

10. Help you achieve your goals

If you are interested in physical activity that helps you stay healthy or lose weight, yoga is for you. In addition to being a physical exercise, however, it is also an activity that fortifies the spirit and increases willpower.

The moments of concentration and meditation offered by yoga will encourage you to move forward. In addition, they will increase the ability to wait patiently for the results of your efforts.

With which positions can you lose weight?

Yoga strengthens muscles, improves flexibility and breathing, and generally helps you feel better. Yoga for those who are overweight is highly recommended because, without involving excessive physical exertion or high intensity, it offers good results.

WHAT IS CHAIR YOGA?

We will not talk about Utkatasana, the infamous chair pose but about practicing Chair Yoga. ***A practice that is in all respects a real Yoga session or an activity to be included every now and then during the many hours spent in the office or in front of the computer.***

Most people spend at least 8 hours sitting in the office, going out to get into the car and sitting again for the journey home, at home they sit at the table and maybe after dinner they spend the evening sitting on the sofa watching TV.

This means that we sit for 10-12 hours a day with serious consequences for our health. In addition to causing fatigue in the neck and shoulders, back, hips and legs, sitting for long periods of time increases the risk of diabetes, increased cholesterol, and postural and muscle problems, just to name a few.

Training sessions in the gym or in the Yoga center are useful for moving the body (if you go there, the registration alone does not lead to significant improvements!) but often they are not enough to balance all those hours sitting.

Sit, sit, sit!

The best thing would obviously be to sit down less, but if this is not really possible, we can increase our "daily movement" with a simple Yoga practice on the chair, so that we can move the spine without even moving from the workplace.

While Yoga in the middle of the workday might seem crazy, it's actually a time-effective way to combat some of these health risks.

After many hours of sitting, your back starts to ache and your neck stiffens, you try to find a more comfortable position on the chair but after a while nothing seems to improve your situation, the pain persists and you spend the rest of the afternoon with contracted muscles.

What you can do is take a few minutes to practice some simple Yoga Asanas on the chair.

Not only do some targeted poses strengthen your core and spine, but they can also help you open your lungs, activate your breath, focus your mind, and stretch your entire body without ever leaving your chair completely.

Greetings To the Sun on The Chair

This simple sun salutation is good for the

SPINE, ABDOMINAL AND BACK MUSCLES

To begin,

sit tall with your feet flat on the floor,

your buttocks well supported in the middle of the chair, and your back straight.
Inhale, bringing your arms above your head.

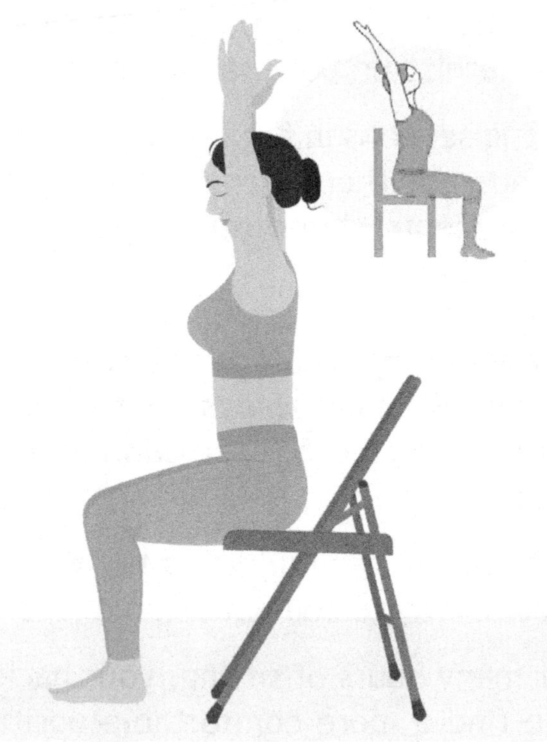

When you are in this position remember to tighten your abdominalsso as not to arch your back too much and to keep your shoulders relaxed.

It is the arms that rise, not the shoulders!

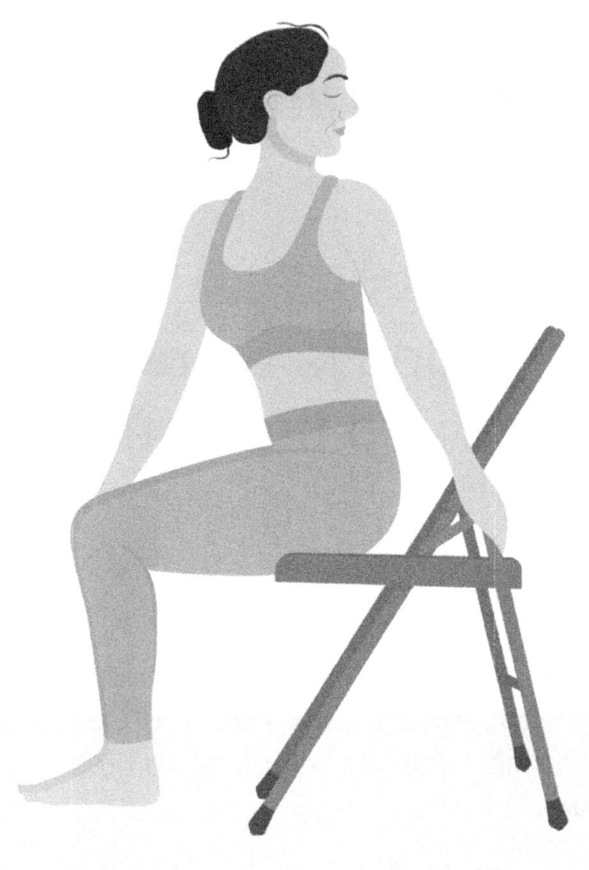

As you exhale, lower your arms
and turn your torso to the leftopening your chest wide,
bring your right hand to your left knee
and your left arm behind the back of thechair.
Inhale again,
bringing your body back to centerand arms up,
then repeat on the right side.

Repeat the sequence eight to ten times.

Adho Mukha Svanasana on the Chair

The down-looking dog is a great way to stretchthe back and the entire back of the body.

In the office, however, seeing you place your hands on the ground and bring your butt upwards under the noses of colleagues could be embarrassing, this version instead turns out to be much more discreet and just as effective.

Start by moving to the back of the chair,place your hands on the backrest, shoulder-width apart.

Bring your feet back until your torso is parallel to the floor.

While holding the asana, think about activating the abdominals and pelvic floor, rotating the coccyx upwards and the iliac crests downwards. As you stretch your back, try to open your shoulderswell by closing your shoulder blades.

Hold the position for eight to 10 breaths

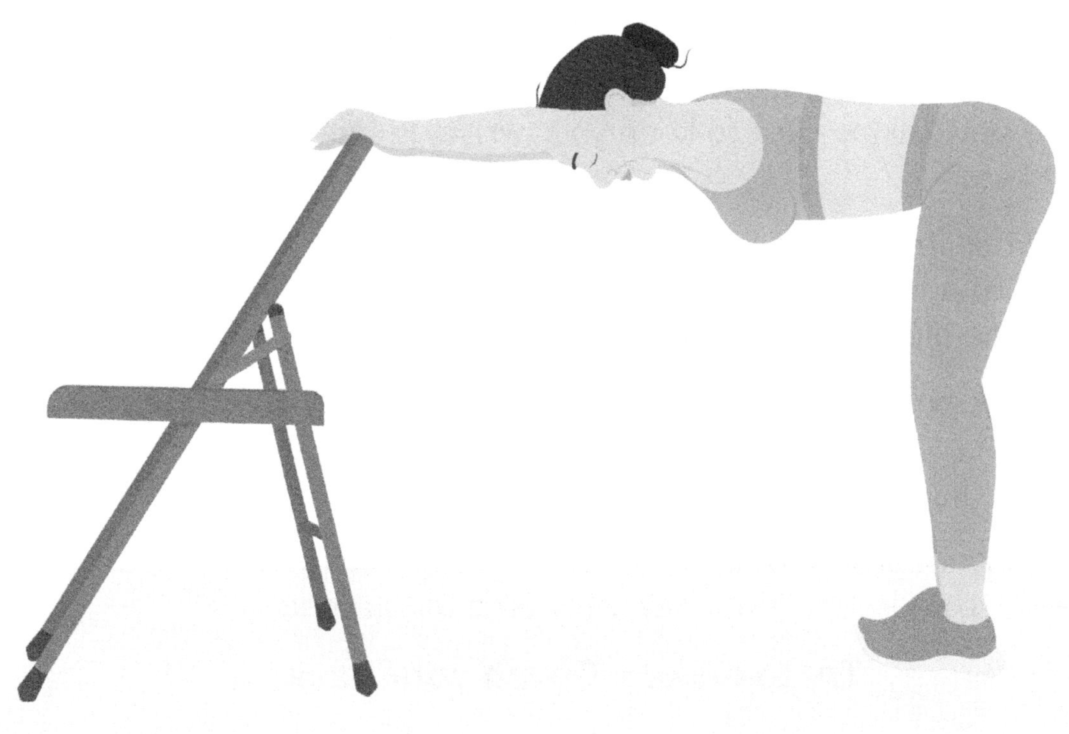

Marjari Asana in the Chair

Marjari Asana, or the cat pose, is usually performed inquadrupedal but also this asana can be performed standing by placing the hands on the seat of the chair.

Move to the front of a chair without armrests and place your hands on the seat,taking care to keep your wrists in line under your shoulders.

Bring your feet in line under the pelvis, no more forward nor backward and nottoo far apart or together. The ankles should be below the hips.

From this position, exhale, and try to form a hump with the back, closing theabdominals and bringing the navel upwards and the gaze towards the knees.

Breathing in, push your buttocks upwards, stretch your back, also looking up andpushing the navel towards the ground.

Try to make a C with your back.

Move slowly and gently, and only when you feel your back warming, try to make each step deeper, more intense, alwayslistening to your body and avoiding pain.

Repeat 15-20 times, always tying the movement with your breath.

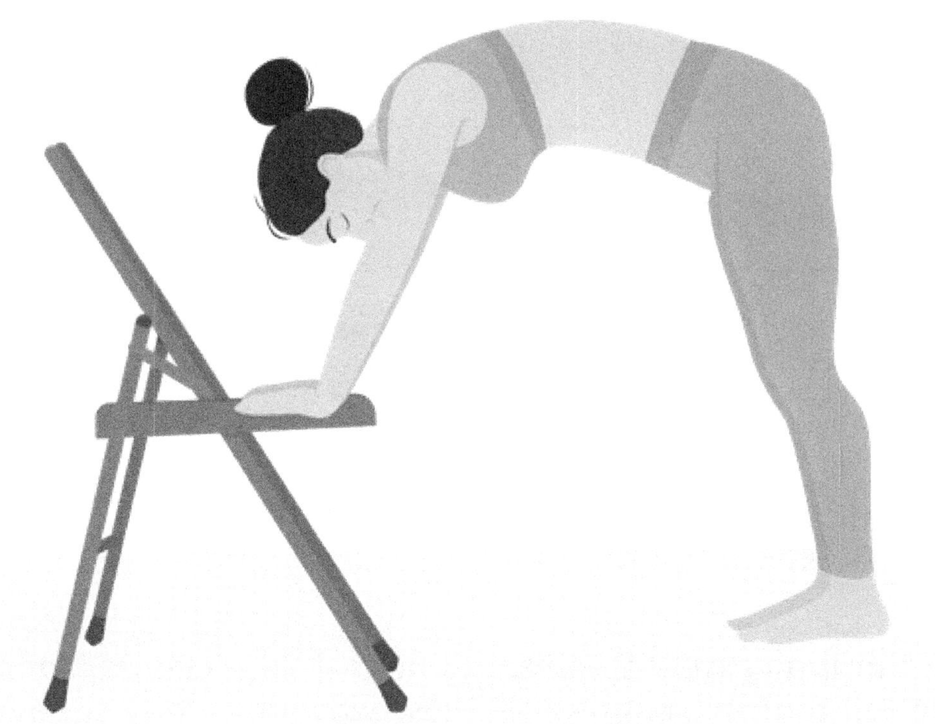

Yoga for everyone

Yoga on a chair is an excellent variant to normal Yoga classes, not only for those who are forced to sit too long, but also for those who are elderly or have motor problems, for those who are overweight or have been sedentary for many years.
Practicing the Asanas with the support of a chair can help to start moving the body, regain elasticity and strength and prepare it for performing bodyweight Yoga sessions in the future.

CHAPTER 1 ASANA ON THE CHAIR FOR BEGINNERS

Chair yoga has been shown to improve flexibility and mobility in those

who havedifficulty moving freely. It helps us to use the mind-body connection, which becomes more and more important with age.

Chair yoga has been shown to benefit overweight people by helping them lose weight.

Who is Yoga Chair really for?

Everyone. We hear a lot that yoga is for everyone. But what about those who have disabilities or who cannot move in certain ways?

Chair yoga is actually for everyone. Even if you have a few extra pounds, you can do chair yoga! Everyone can also do yoga.

When it comes to yoga, it's best to keep it simple. You definitely don't want to use a chair with wheels and the armrests can also cause problems if you want to move your arms or legs.

Look for a simple but sturdy folding chair. Using one that has a rigid seat and back is ideal; in this case, less is more.

6 Major Benefits of Chair Yoga

1. Improve flexibility

Many people find flexibility one of those things that goes away with age. But in reality, flexibility takes practice.

If you do nothing to stretch your muscles, you will obviously lose flexibility. Butif you keep up consistent practice, you can remain flexible throughout your years, not just the "early" years.

Anyone who has difficulty touching their toes, turning their head to one side or the other of the body, will benefit significantly from chair yoga.

2. Improve strength

Chair yoga strengthens all those little stabilizing muscles that we use every day.The muscles and tendons around the ankles, shoulders and hips will be engagedat some point in a chair yoga session.

These muscles are the ones that will protect you from injury if you fall or makea misstep. A stronger body is able to resist and heal quicker from injuries.

3. Increase body awareness

The yoga chair forces you to bring your awareness into your body. As you deepenyour breath and slow down your movements, you will begin to train your brain to focus more on your body.

Having body awareness promotes a powerful unity between body and mind, conscious interaction with the world around us, and a greater sense of self. Chair yoga encourages deep breathing techniques, which helps you tune into what's going on in the body and stay present.

4. Reduces stress, promotes relaxation

   We all have to take the time to slow down every now and then. The yoga chair is perfect for anyone who is stressed out, overworked or just needs a few minutesaway from the hustle and bustle of everyday life.

   When we give ourselves the opportunity to take a break, even for just a few minutes, we regain mental clarity and relaxation. Being relaxed and calming down leads to feelings of happiness and well-being. And everyone can benefit from it!

5. Meet new people

   Young or old, we all benefit greatly from socialization. Chair yoga is a great wayto meet like-minded people from all walks of life. This is especially useful for the elderly or those who are unable to go out a lot.

6. Pain management

   Pranayama can help with pain management.

   We learn how to respond rather than react to our emotions, making it easier to deal with difficult situations like chronic pain or even just moments of stress.

   Mindfulness and attention to the breath simply reminds us keep breathing whenthe going gets tough.

   We've collected six different chair yoga poses to get you started.

Cat and Cow

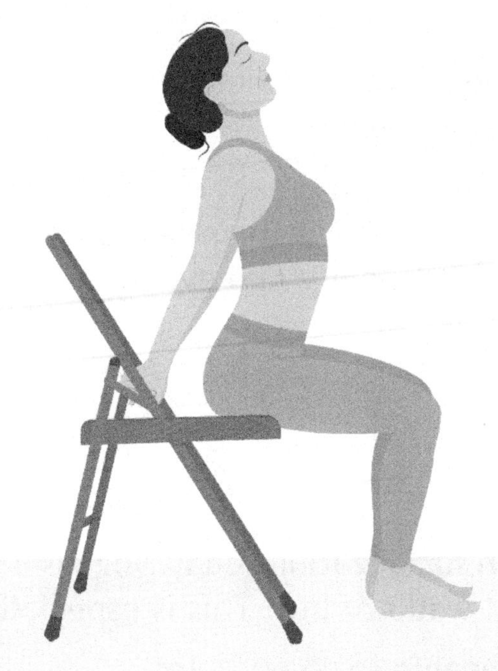

Benefits: The Cat and Cow Pose is aclassic yoga pose that helps build the connection between the lower spine and pelvis, as well as the upper spine and shoulders. Fortunately, it can easily be done in a chair!

Sit close to the edge of the chair. During an inhalation, slowly arch your back, bringing your chest forward and pulling your tailbone and shoulders back.

To exhale, bend the back forward, pulling the chest back and pulling the tailbone and shoulders forward.

Repeat 3 to 5 times

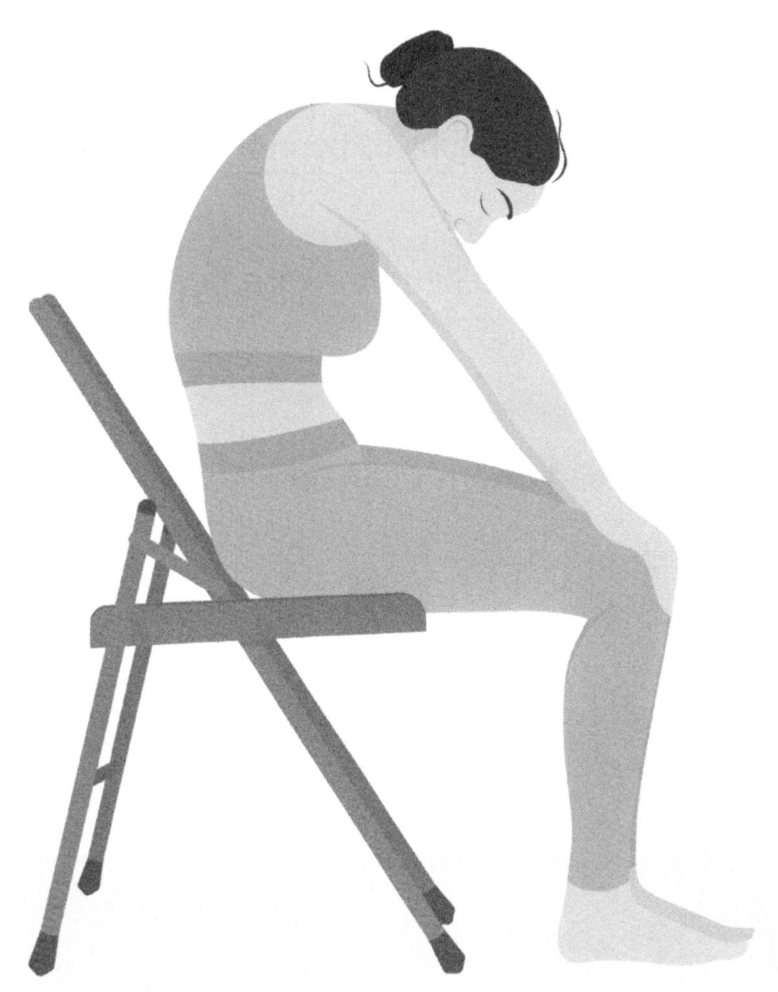

Forward Bend

Benefits: here's another great way to stretch yourhamstrings and prevent hip and lower back pain!

This time we stay behind the chair.

Place both hands on the shoulder-width backrest

and walk back slightly until the torso begins to bend towards the floor.

Maintain a slight bend in your knees

and keep your back very straight as you bend forward.Keep some weight on the chair for support.

As you inhale,

press into the back of the chair and return to an upright position.

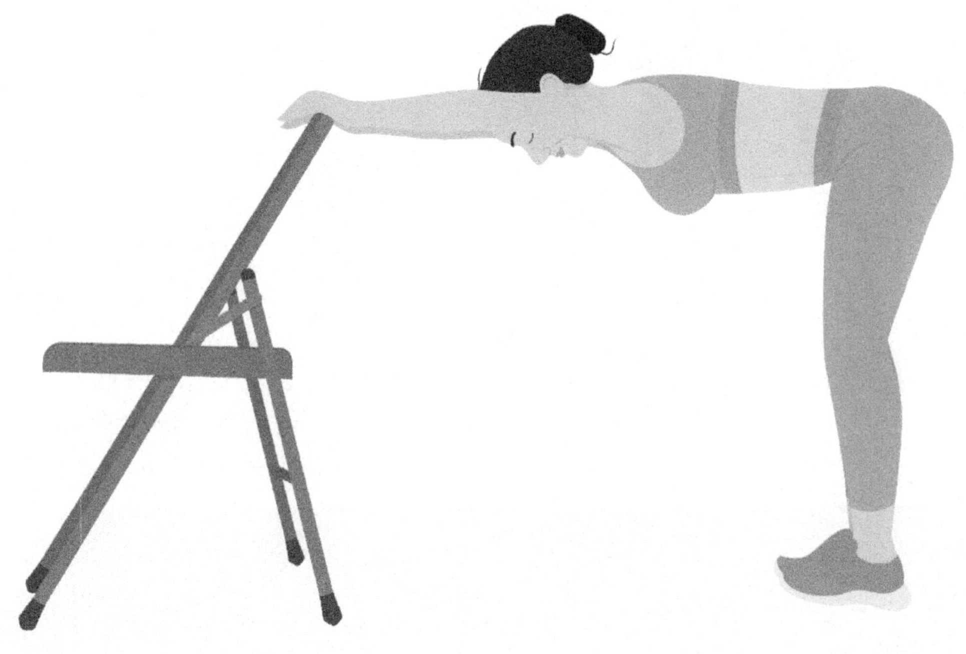

Eagle pose

This position works perfectly to help improve balance and, at the same time, works on the thighs, legs and arms.

This means that it is perfect for strengthening the abdominal muscles and hips.

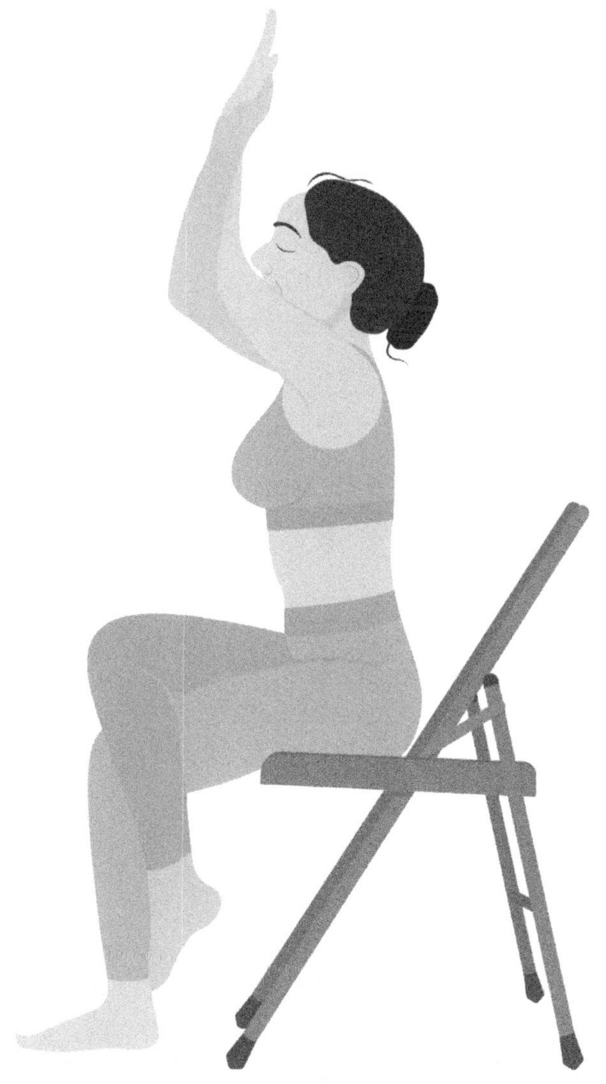

Cross your left leg over your right leg so that the knees are close together.

If mobility allows, move your right foot slightly forwardand wrap your left toes around your right calf.

Cross your left elbow over your right elbow and keep your arms at an angle of 90 degrees,with your fingers pointing towards the ceiling.

Hold the pose here

or experiment with taking the weight off the chair and balancing yourself.

Warrior I pose

Benefits: This is a great way to use a chair to make a classic strength-building pose more accessible.

Sit towards the left half of the seat

and bend your right leg at 90 degrees to the front of the seat.

Bend your left leg, keeping slightly at the

knee.Press the ball of

the left foot to the

floor, heel up.

Press firmly on both feet

and try to lift your weight off the chair.

If the pose is comfortable,

raise your hands up and hold there.

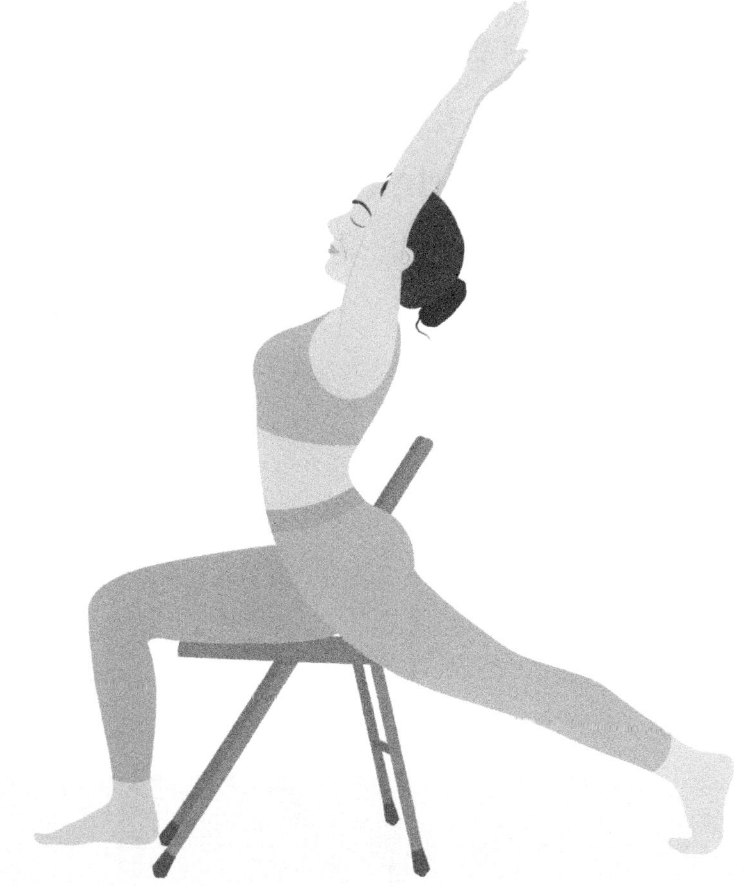

Repeat on both sides

Warrior II Pose

Advantages: Just like Warrior One, Warrior Two can also be modified for a chair.

Sit towards the left side of the chair and open your right leg at a 90-degree angle to the front of the chair.

Open your left leg and stretch it to the left,keeping only a slight bend in the knee. Keep your chest open forward.

Press firmly on both feet and try to lift the weight off the chair.

If the pose is comfortable, bring your hands together and stretch your arms to opposite sides of the room.

Repeat on both sides.

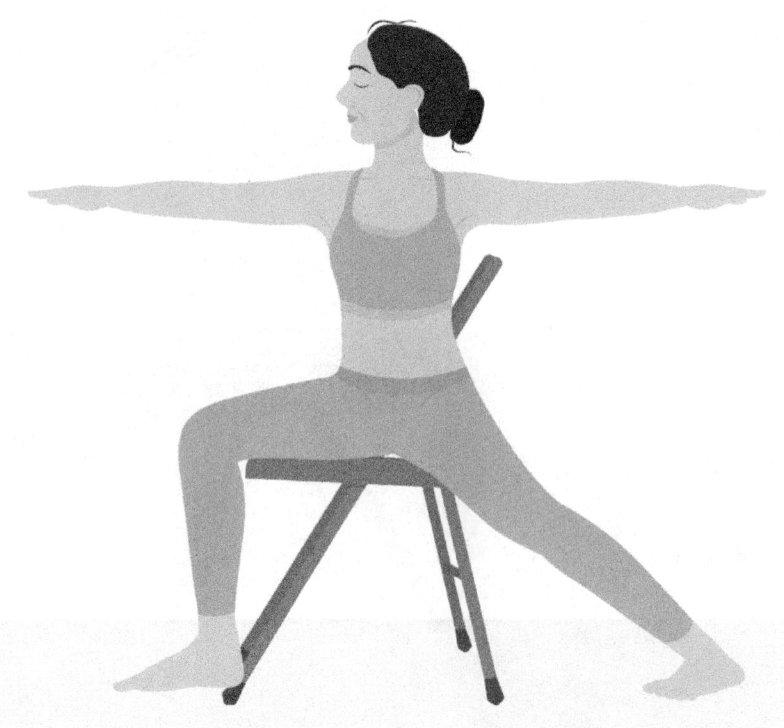

Yoga Pigeon Pose

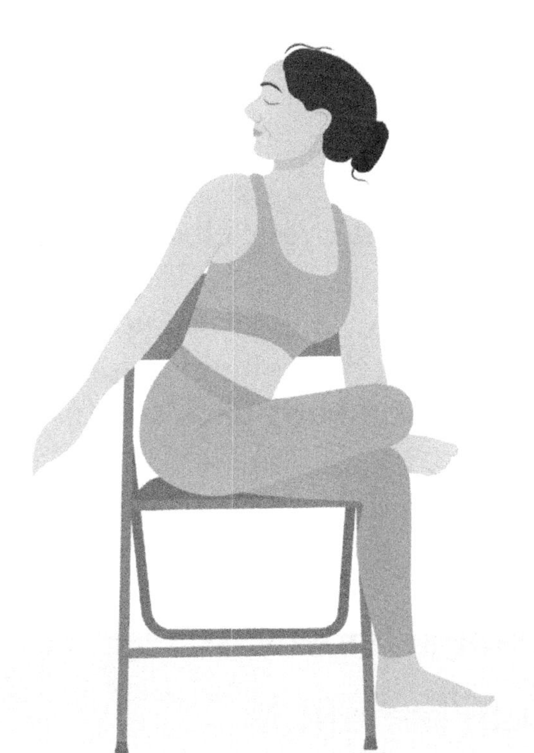

A yoga posture that helps release tension in the musclesof the lower back, hips, and hamstrings.

In addition, regular practice of this asana is helpfulin opening the hips, reducing sciatica symptoms and relieving hip and knee pain.

Sit towards the left side of the chair and bend your right leg at a 90-degree angle to the front of the chair.

Rotate your chest to the right at a 45-degree angle from the front of the chair.

Bring your right leg into the chair, closing the joint by half. Reach your left leg back and press your toes to the floor, heel up.

This pose may not be suitable for people with knee pain orvery stiff hips.

Rotation of the elbow

Benefits: This simple stretch can help relieve shoulder and upper back stiffness from prolongedperiods of sitting.

Sit tall in your chair.

Place your fingertips on your shoulders and relax your elbows.

Bring your elbows forward so they are close but not touching.
BEGIN THE ROTATION by lifting them towards the ceiling,keeping the head elevated. Separate the elbows and move the elbows back and forth,completing the rotation.
As the elbows separate, the shoulder blades should come together.

Perform this movement as slowly as possiblefor maximum benefit.

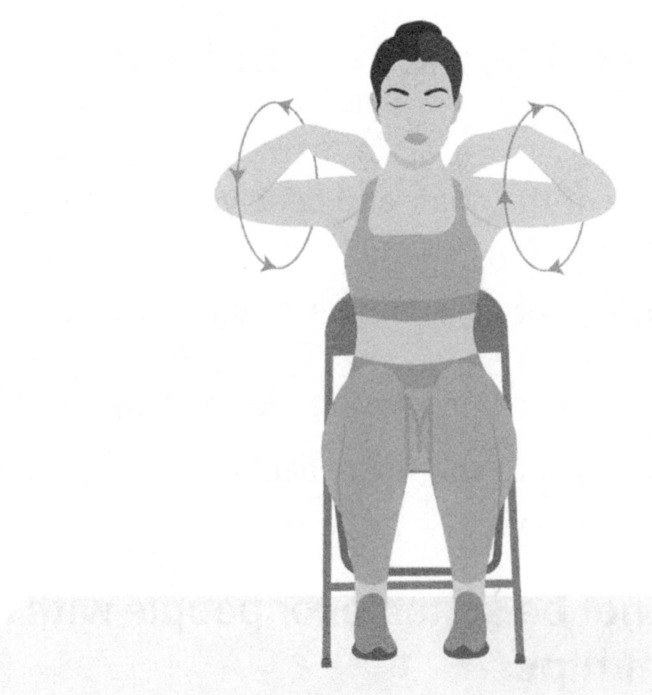

Hip stretches

Benefits: This exercise is great for relieving tensionin the hips and lower back, as well as relieving sciatic nerve irritation.

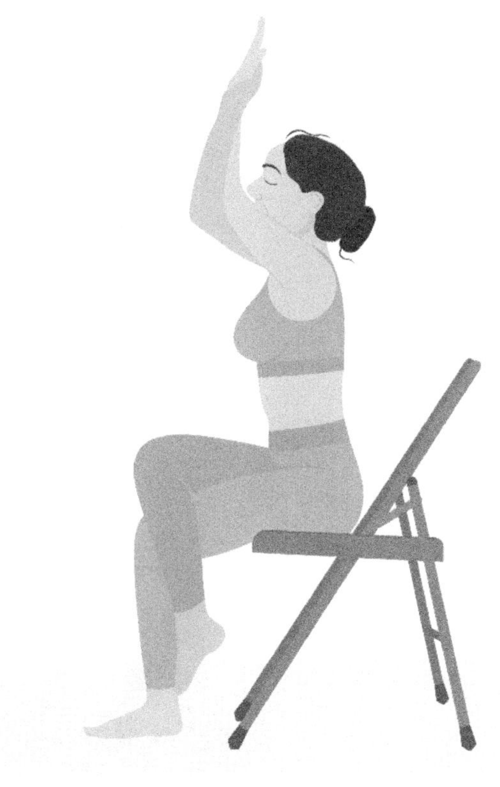

Start by sitting forward, towards the edge ofthe chair.

Place the right heel on the left knee. The knee will fall to the right side. Start gently bending forward until you feel astretch in your right hip joint.

To deepen, gently press the knee down with the elbows. If there is tension or pressure in the knee, back off a little.

For maximum benefit, repeat the pose asecond time before continuing.

Make sure you repeat on the other side.

Sit lightly on the right side of the chair, sothat your right hip releases slightly from the
chair. Cross your right leg over your left so that your knees are close to touching.Grab your right foot with your left hand.
Keep this foot elevated as you bend forward, deepening the stretch.

Repeat the pose a second time before continuing and be sure to repeatit on the other side.

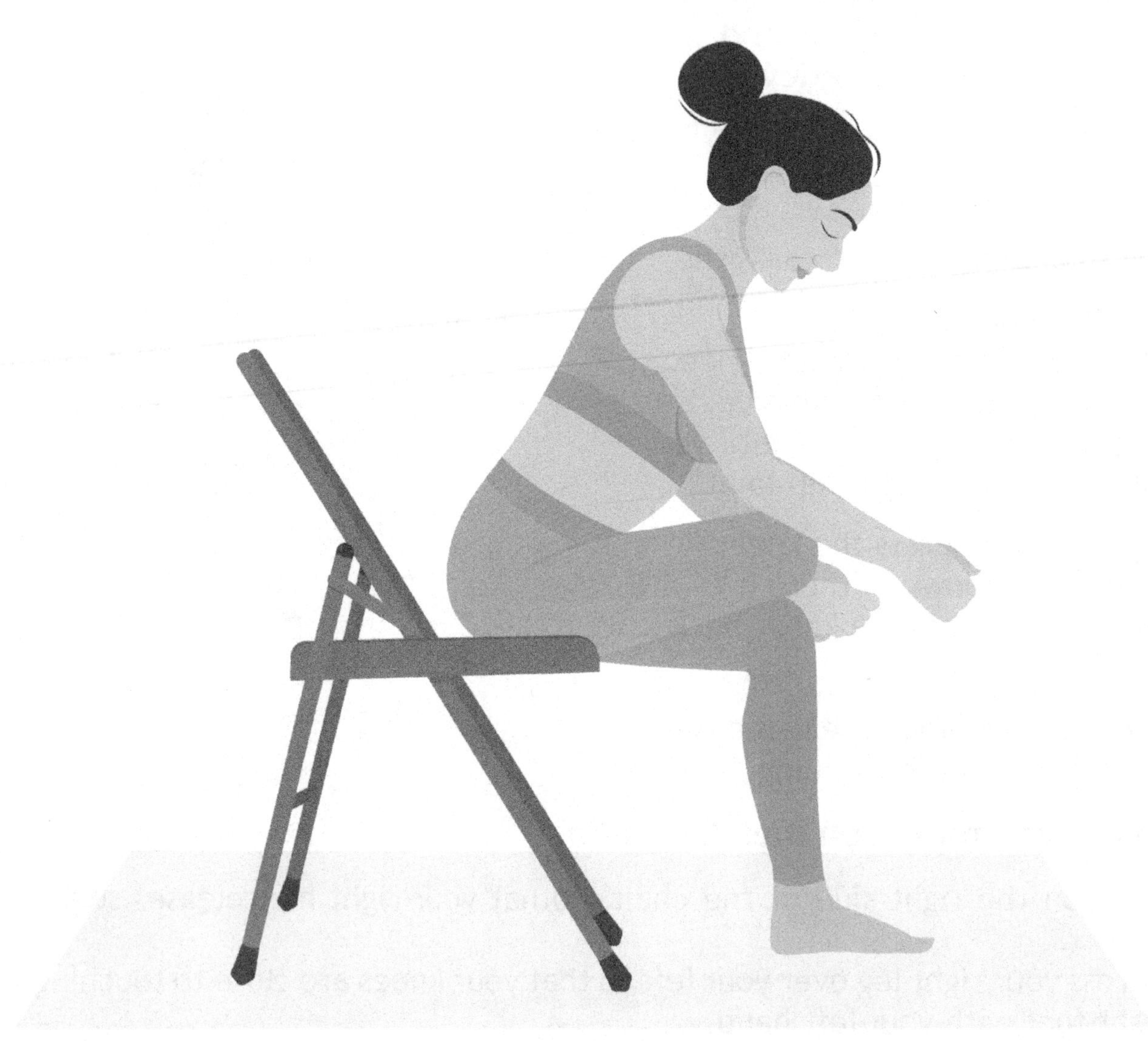

Rotations of the ankle

Benefits: We often neglect the mobility and strengthof our feet, but this is a key factor in maintaining mobility and independence as we age. These exercises can help.

Place the right heel on the left knee in a "four"

position.The knee will fall to the right side.

Hold the right ankle on the left thigh with the right hand and place each of the fingers of the left hand between the toes of the right foot.

Use your left hand to guide the foot in a slow rotation throughout its range of motion.

Make sure you move both clockwise and counterclockwise.

Repeat on both sides.

Straighten your right leg, keeping your foot in the air.

Start by flexing the foot so that the toes turn towards the body and perform aslow rotation of the ankle.

Perform this movement both clockwise and counterclockwise.

Repeat on both sides.

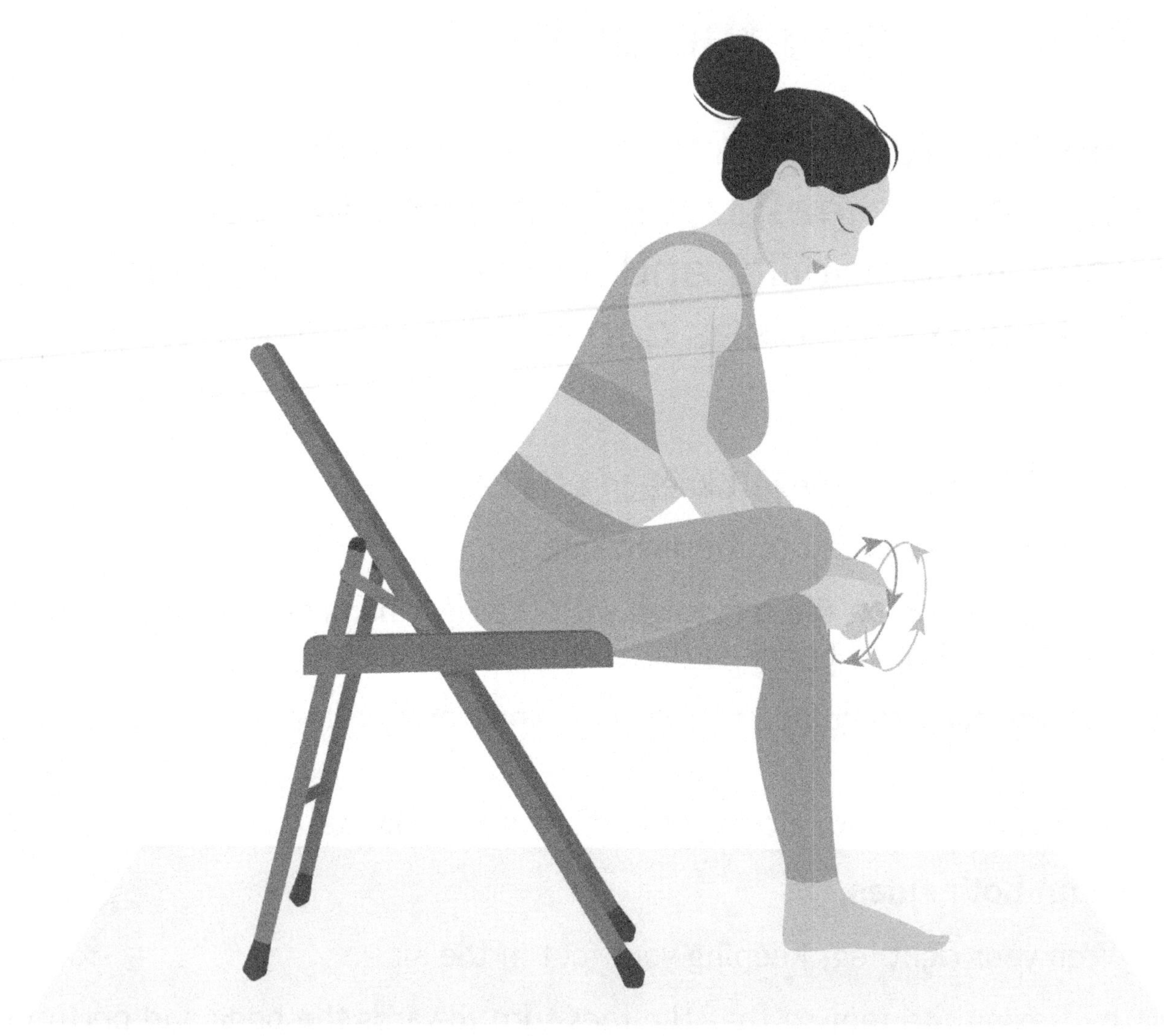

Knee reinforcement

Benefits: knee discomfort is a common complaint in aging populations. As we age, it is very important todevelop strength around the knee joint by performing exercises like these.

Start by placing a thin but firm pillow between your knees and bring your feet together.

Sit straight and keep your legs at a 90-degree angle.

Press your knees firmly together, squeezing the pillow. **Hold for 15 to 20 seconds and repeat 3 to 5 times.**

Place the pillow under your thighs.

Straighten your right leg, lifting it off the ground. Press the thigh firmly againstthe pillow and flex the toes towards the body. Hold for 10-15 seconds and repeat3 to 5 times.

Repeat with the other leg.

In this exercise we combine the previous two.

Squeeze the pillow between your knees and slowly lift your right leg up until straight, keeping the pillow between your knees.

Hold for 10 seconds and then lower with control.

Repeat on the other side

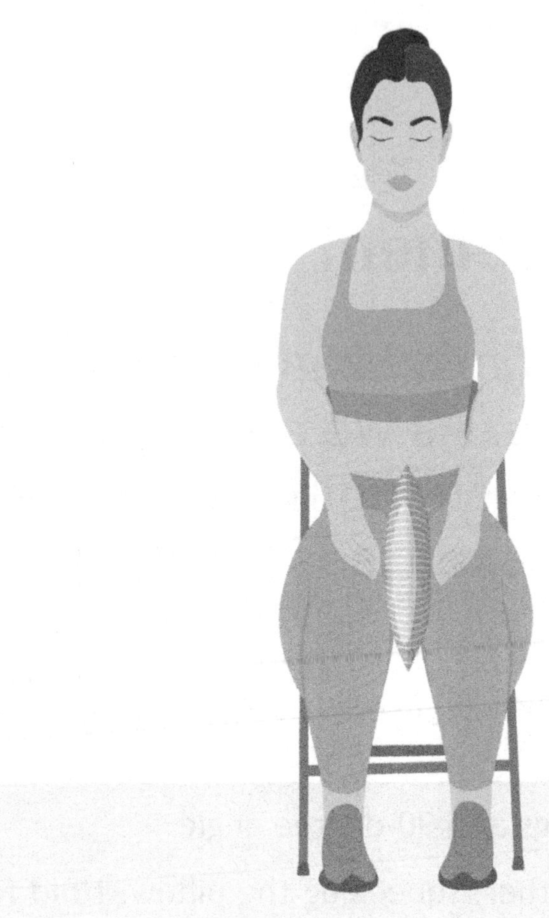

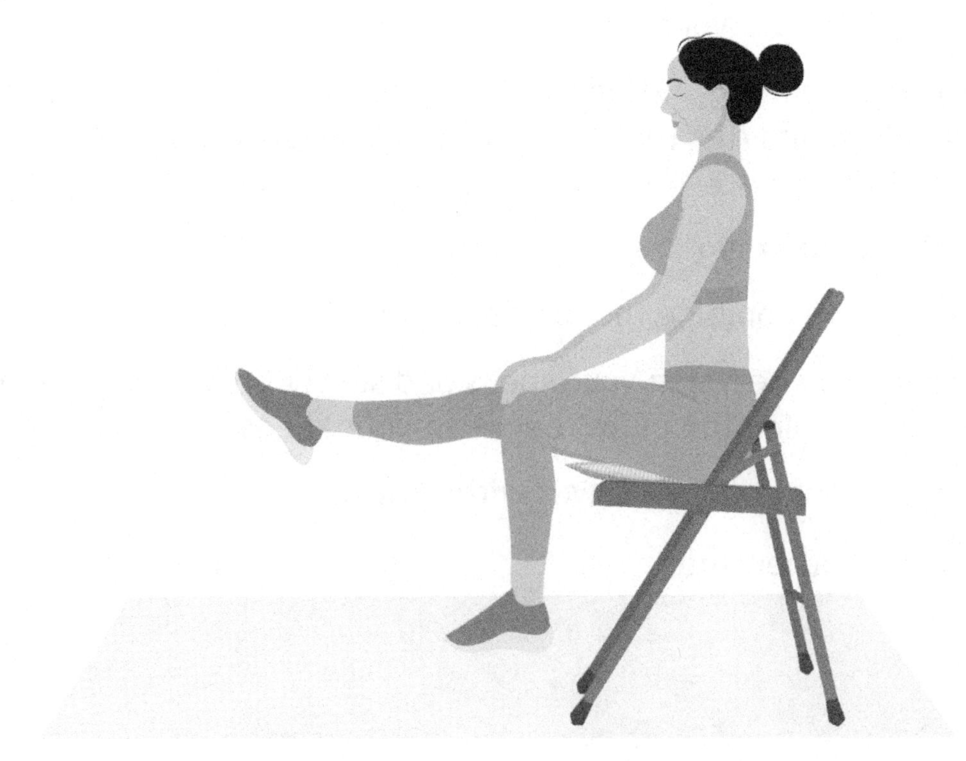

Back bend

Benefits: This exercise can help compensate for back relaxation during periods of prolonged sitting.

Start by sitting on the edge of the chairwith your legs open at 90 degrees. Hold the back of the chair with your arms straight,opening your chest and pushing it forward.

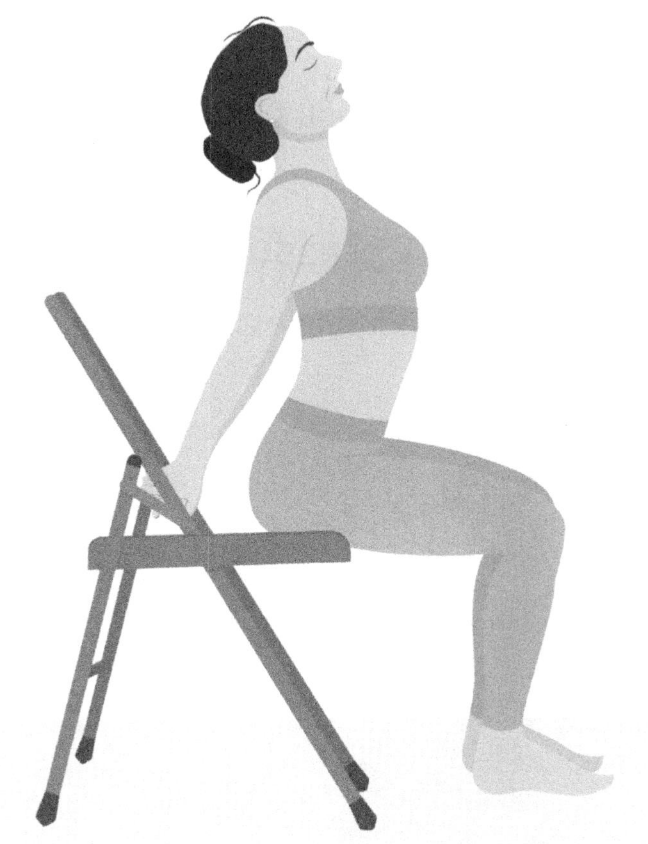

Expand across the front of your body, lifting your chin without throwing your head back.

Let the spine gently arch.

Be careful, if there is any pinch or spasm in the back, back offslightly or release the pose and try again later.

Twisting of the chair

Benefits: twisting through the back can help energize the body and rejuvenate spinal health.

Sit with your legs on the left side of the chair.

Hold each side of the chair back and draw the chest towards the back,turning it to the left.

Use your arms to gently approach the twist.

Make sure you stretch through your spine as you turn, drawing the crown of your head towards the ceiling.

Make sure there is no pinching or pressure in the spine.

This movement should be comfortable and painless.Be aware and kind to yourself.

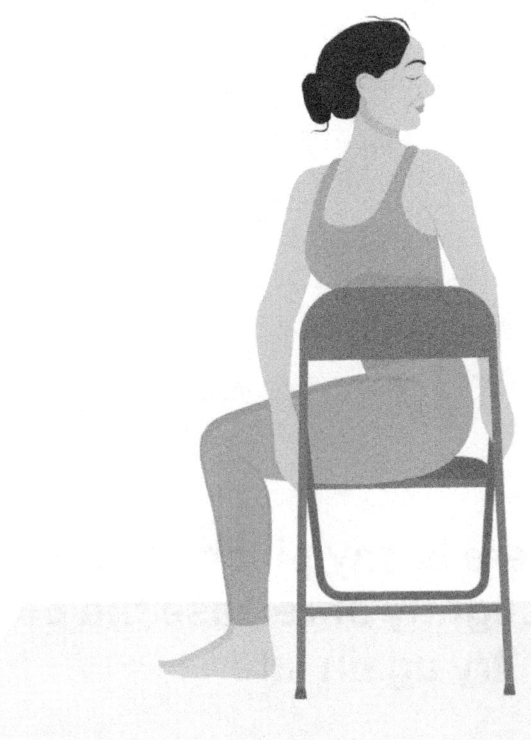

Lateral extension of the chair

Benefits: After twisting or bending the spine, it is important to perform a lateral stretch as well so thatyou have access to the full range of motion of the spine.

Sitting on the edge of the chair.

Spread your knees as far as possible, at a 90-degree angle if possible. Place the right forearm on the right thigh and gently press into the thigh.

Reach your left arm above your head and start reaching for the right side of theroom, stretching the entire left side of your body.

After holding for 3 or 5 breaths, repeat on the other side.

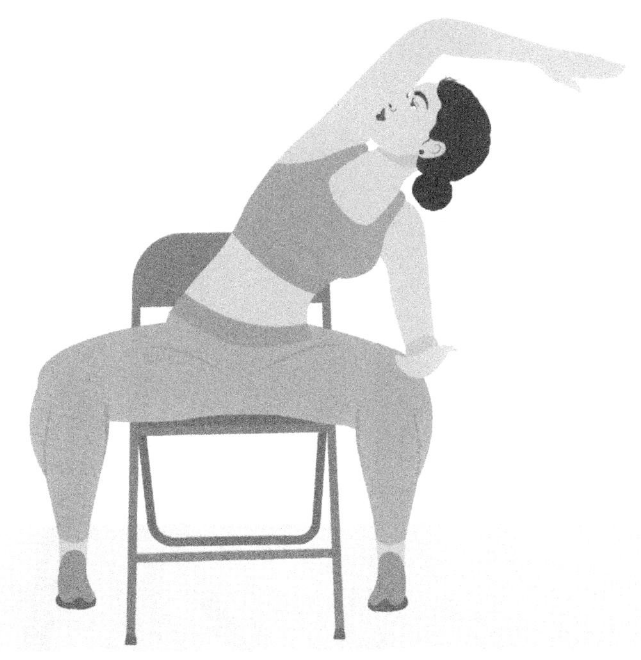

Forearm stretches

Benefits: wrist health is especially important nowadays as we spend more and more time working on a computer or mobile device. Forearmstretches are essential.

Sit towards the back of the chair with your knees apart.

Place your right palm on the chair with your fingers pointing back towards your body, stretching your wrist.

If there is no pain, you can gently press.

If there is pain or pressure, it may be easier to turn the fingers slightly to the right. After repeating for both sides, it can be helpful and slightly deeper to do bothhands at the same time

Hold your right arm in front of your body with your fingers pointing towards the ceiling and use your left hand to gently pull your fingers back.

Hold for 2 to 3 breaths. Rotate your hand so that your fingers are pointing towards the floor and repeat.

Repeat on both sides.

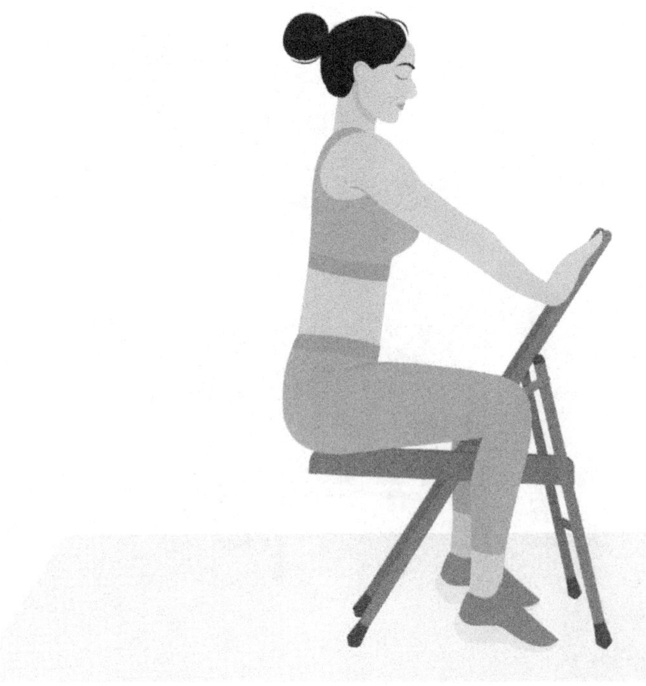

Breathing exercises

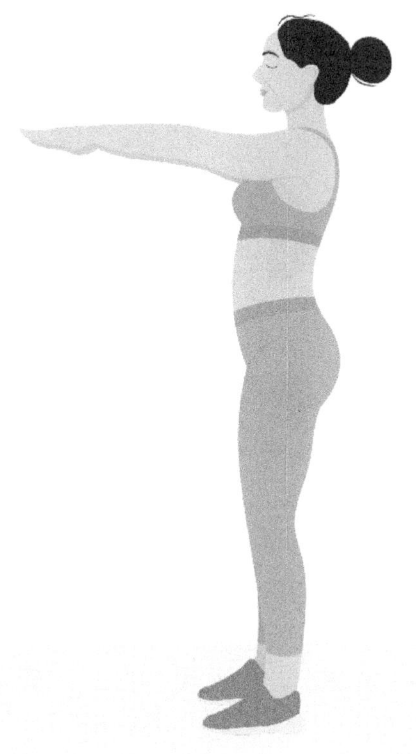

Benefits: in yoga, one of the deepest aspects of the practice is breathing. Fortunately, you can do most of the yogicbreathing exercises perfectly well while sitting in a chair! Here are just a few.

Inhale slowly and deeply. As you inhale, spread yourarms, expanding them across your chest. Keep them straight.

Breathe out with control. As you exhale, bring your arms together, connecting your palms in front of yourbody.

Repeat 5 to 10 times. Start by keeping your arms straight in front of your body,parallel to each other. Inhale slowly and deeply. As you inhale, raise your arms up high.

Breathe out with control. As you exhale, lower your hands to the starting position.

Repeat 5 to 10 times. Start with your arms straight along the sides of your body.Inhale slowly and deeply. As you inhale, raise your hands up in a wide arc, pullingthem away from each other until they meet at the top.

Breathe out with control. Slowly return your hands to their starting position, keeping them straight.

Repeat 5 to 10 times

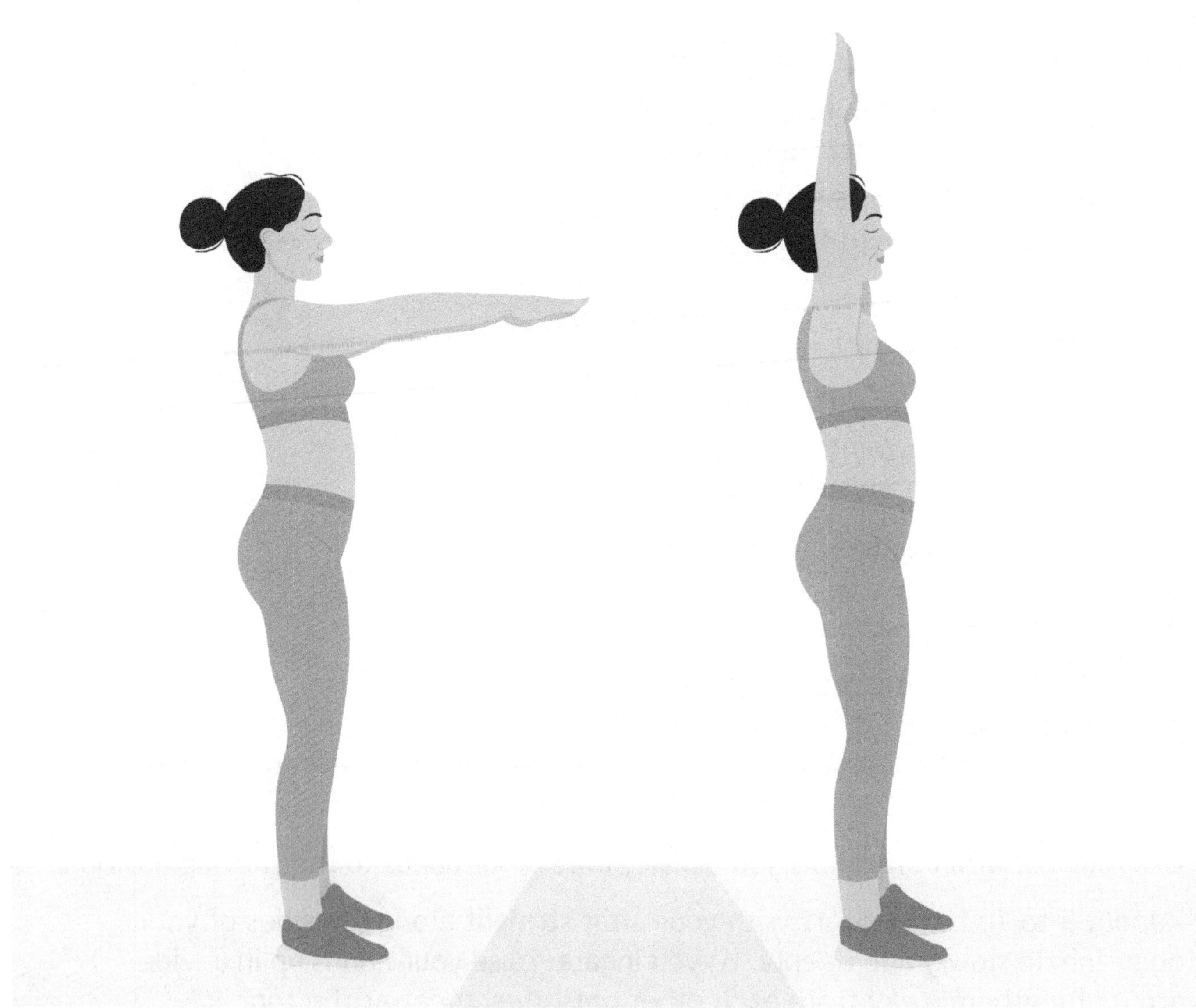

Vertical stretches of the spine

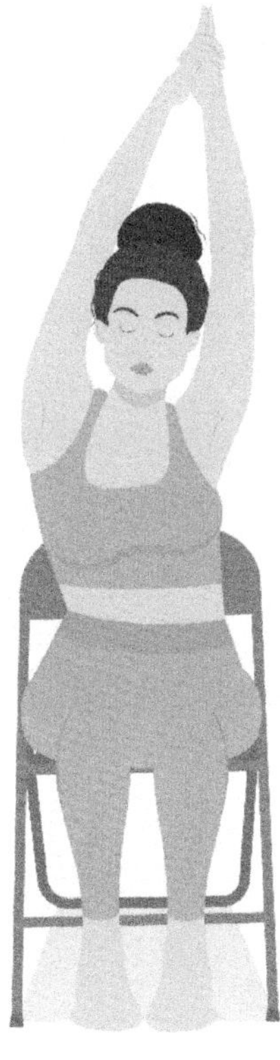

Benefits: this pose helps to stretch the spine, stretch theback muscles, and energize the body.

Start by sitting high at the end of the chair.

Join your hands in a prayer position slightly away from your chest, stretchingacross your wrists.

Press your palms into each other.

On an inhalation raise your hands over your head and reach as high above your head as possible and stretch across the

spine as far as possible.

Try to stretch further with each inhalation. Hold for 3-4 breaths.

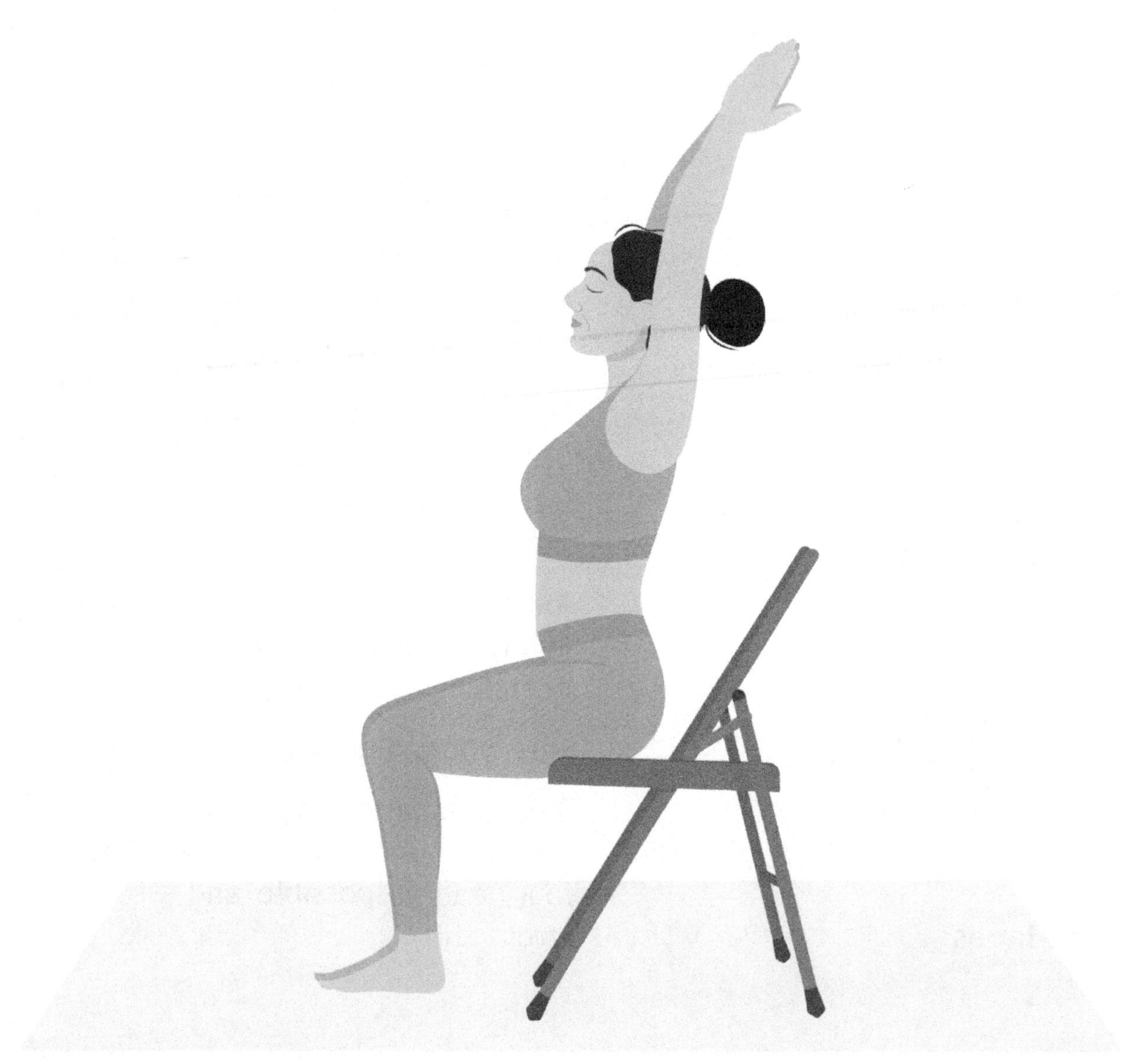

Stretching of the hamstring

Benefits: tight hamstrings are an all-too-common cause of hip and back pain. Regular stretching ofthe hamstrings helps us prevent this pain and maintain the balance and mobility of the legs.

Sit with your legs out to the right side of the chair and your right arm supporting you on the back of the chair. Lift the left foot into the chair and grasp the foot with the left hand.Slowly stretch your leg until you begin to feel a stretch. Keep your back straight.

Repeat on both sides

Sit on the edge of the chair and straighten your left leg,keeping your heel in contact with the floor. Keep the knee slightly bent as you begin to lean forwardwith your back straight. Be careful not to round your spine as you lean forward.

Repeat 2 to 3 times, then repeat on the other side.

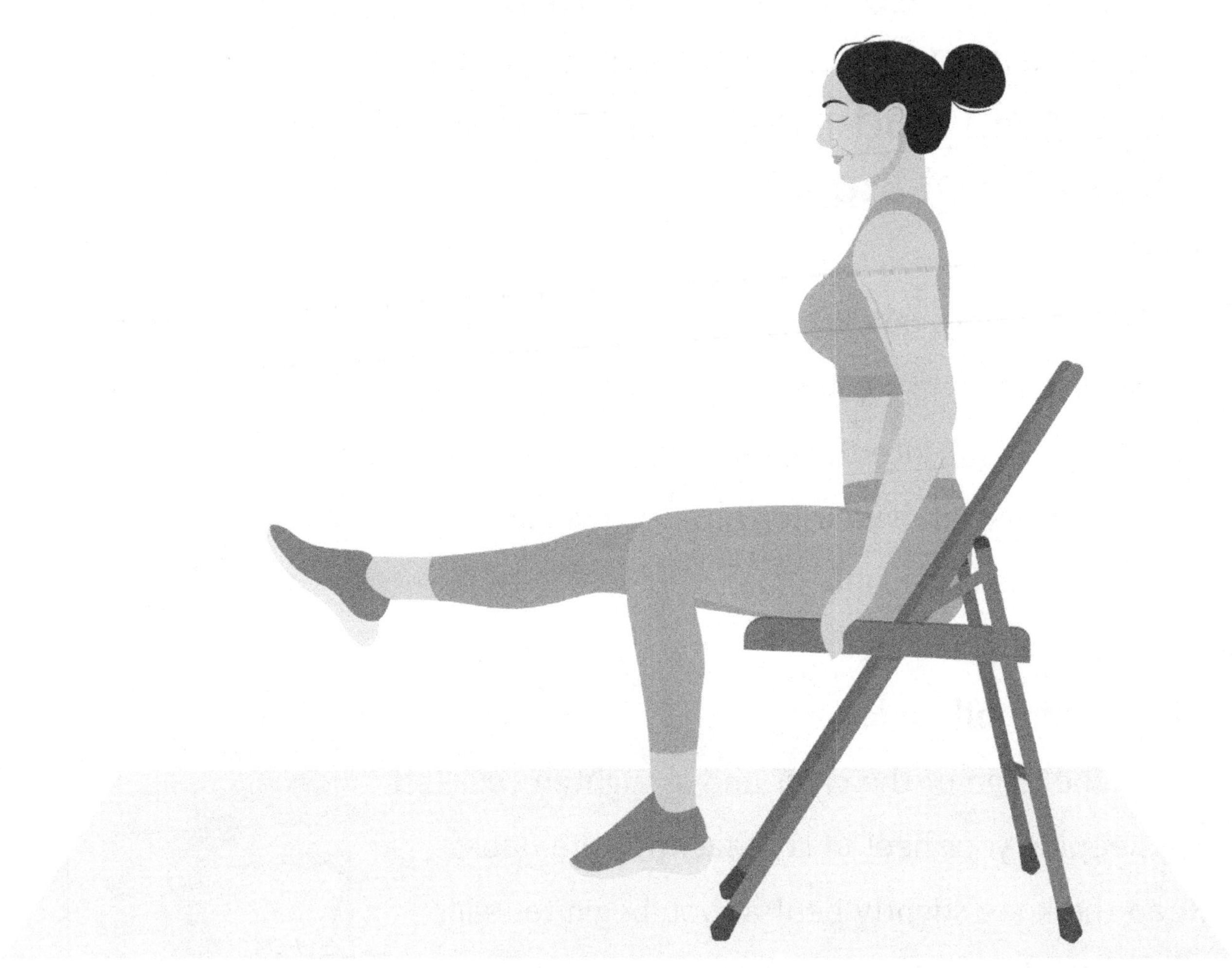

Wrist mobility exercises

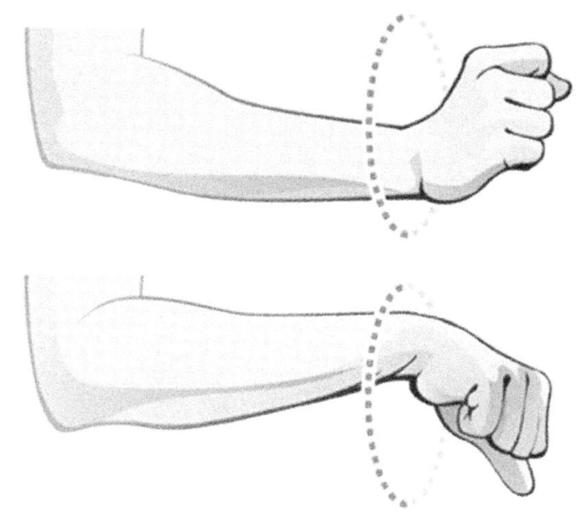

Here are some wristmobility exercises for all the keyboard warriors out there!

Keep your arms straight infront of your body with your hands in fists.

Keep your forearms pointing down and don't bend your elbows. Rotate your wriststhrough their full range of motion, as slowly as possible. **Repeat 10 times clockwise and 10 times counterclockwise.**

Keep your arms straight in front of your body with your hands outstretched, palms towards the floor. Without moving your arms or rotating your forearms, move your fingers as far to the left as possible, keeping your palms facing the floor. Then, move them to the right before returning to the first position. **Repeat 10 times.**

Keep your arms straight in front of your body with your hands outstretched, palms towards the floor. Without moving your arms or rotating your forearms reach your fingertips towards the ceiling. Then, reach your fingertips towards the floor before returning to the first position.

Repeat 10 times.

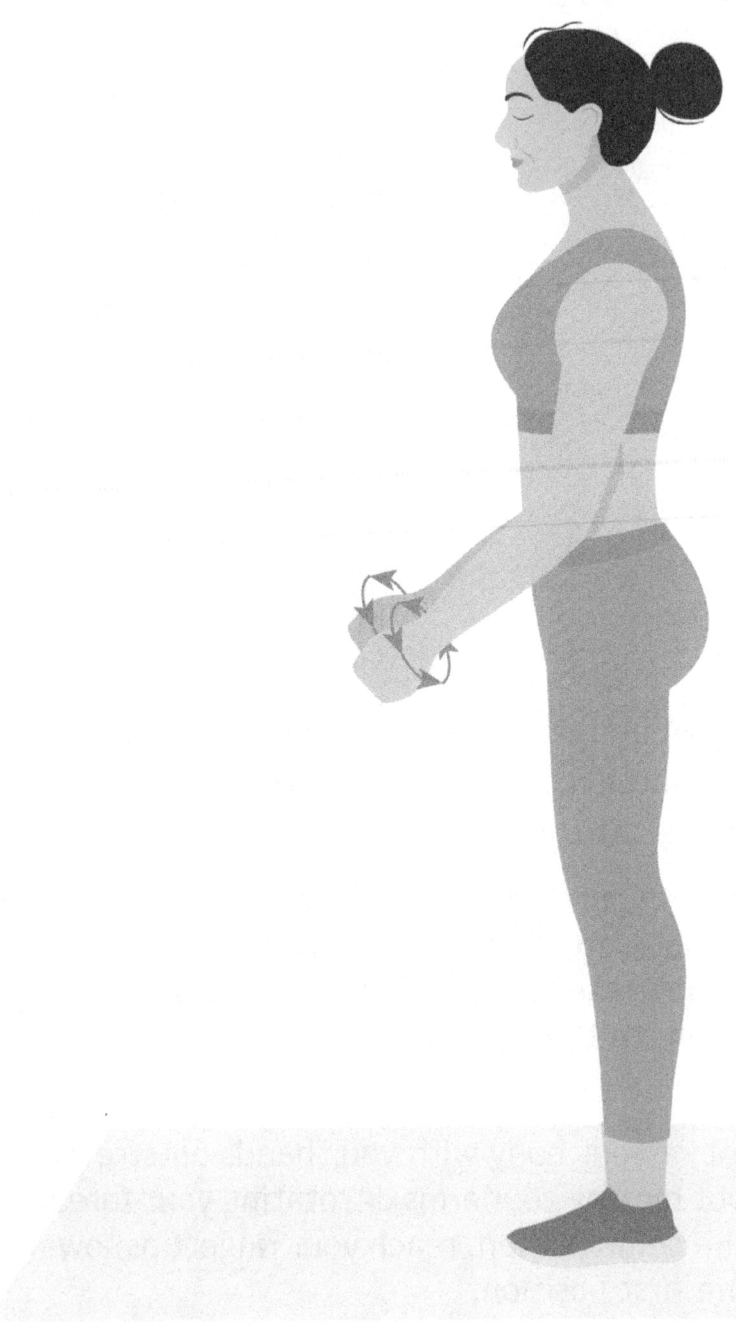

Scapular movement

Benefits: building flexibility in the shoulder blades can help prevent sagging when sitting for long periods of time. Here is an exercise that can help.

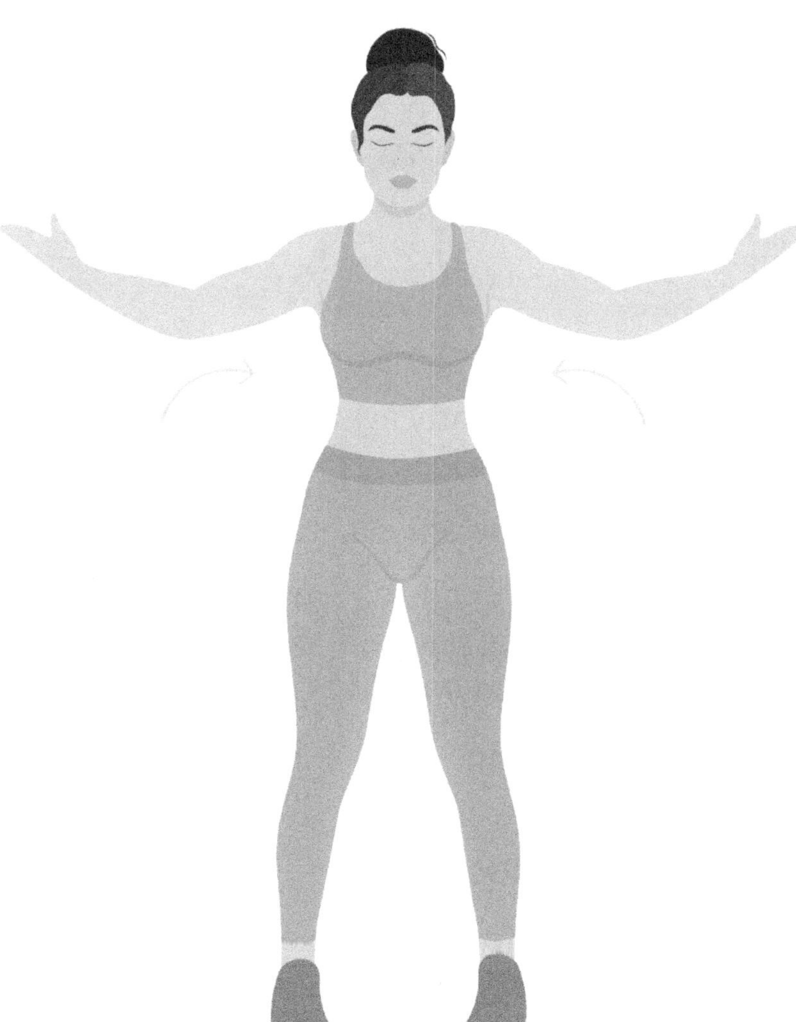

During an inhalation,open your arms,

keeping your elbows only slightly bent.

Draw the shoulders back and shoulder blades together.

As you exhale, bring your elbow in front of your body, rounding your upper back.Draw shoulders forward and shoulder blades away from each other.

Repeat 10 times.

Surya Namaskar in a Chair

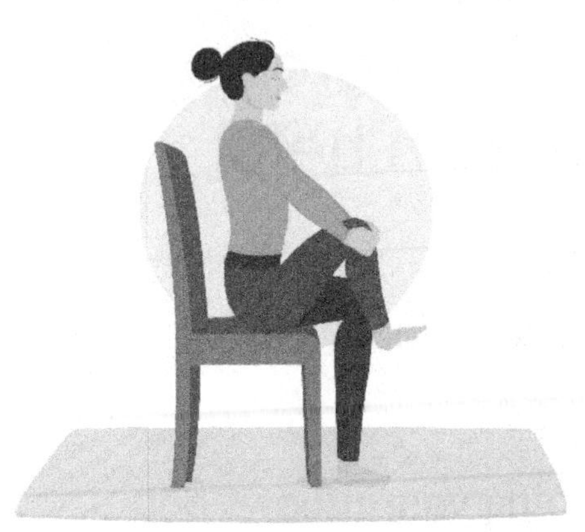

Start with the back ofthe chair behind you.Supporting your backwith a pillow in your lower back can be helpful, and keeping a pillow under your buttocks can also help.

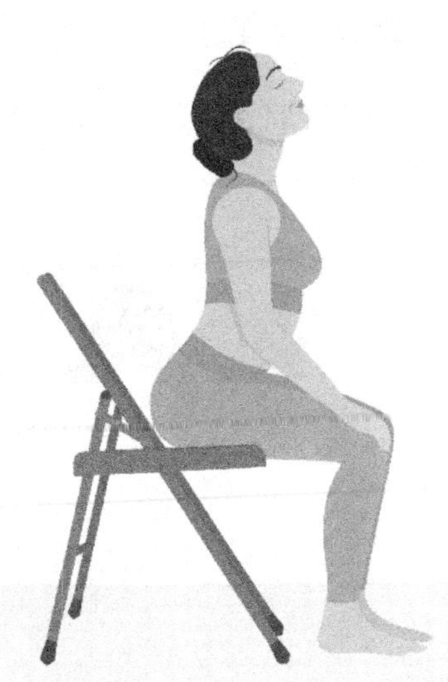

Inhaling, raise your arms above your head and lean gently against the back of the chair, being careful not to drop your neck too far back.

As you exhale, keeping your back straight, slowly wrap your torso over your legs, sliding your hands along your shins.

Inhaling, slide your hands back and return to a sitting position, pulling your right knee towards your chest. Lean back on the chair and open it across your chest.

Exhale around the back and bring the head closer to the knee, lowering the shoulders.

Release your right leg. Repeat on the other side.

After both sides are completed, stretch your arms forward and lean against the back of the chair, do another forward bend, go back and do a final back bend, and come back to standing with your hands in a prayer position.

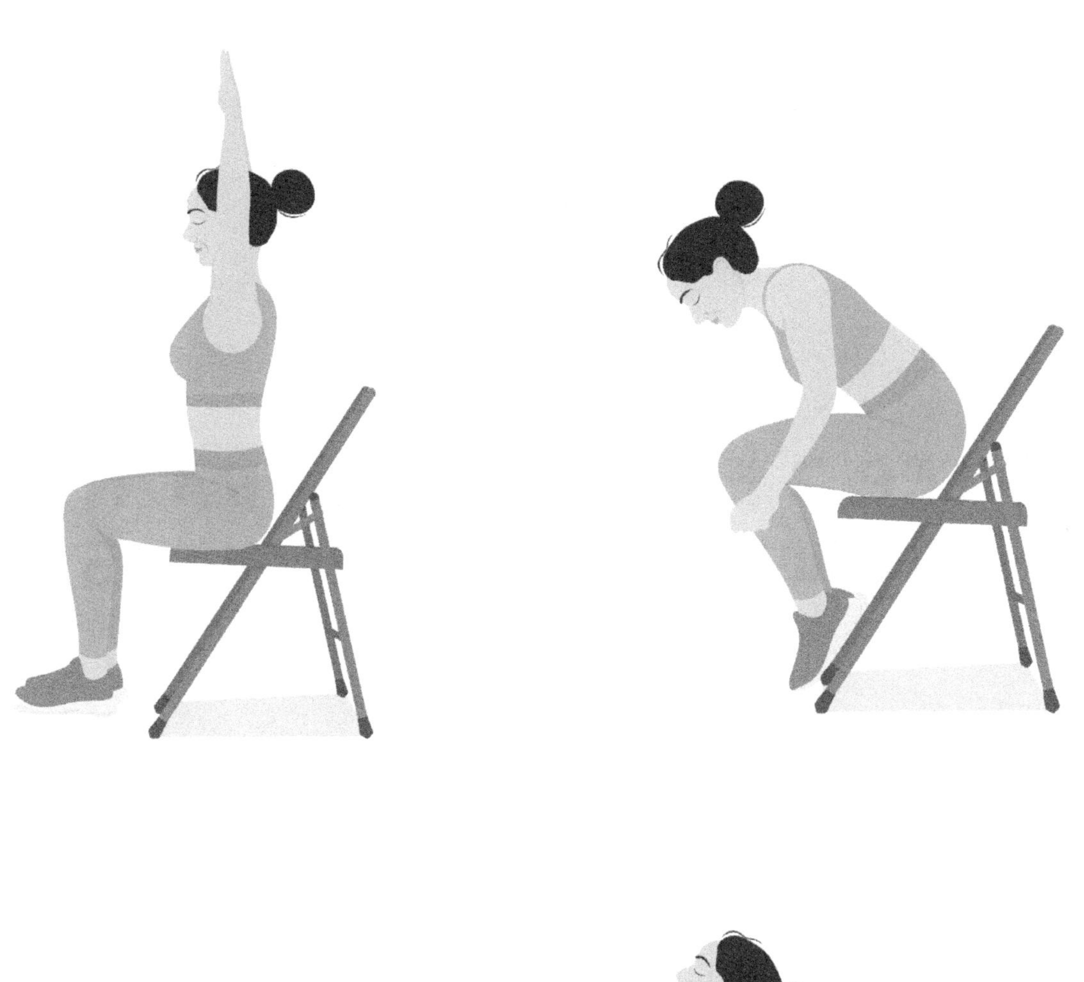

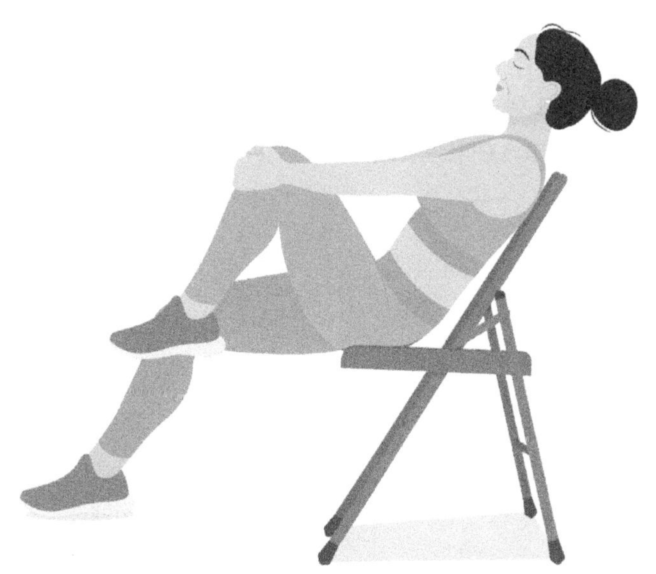

CHAPTER 2 EXAMPLE OF TRAINING SESSIONS FOR BEGINNERS

Chair yoga is a form of yoga therapy developed by Lakshmi Voelker-Binder in 1982. It is practiced while sitting in a chair or standing, using the chair as a support. If you spend many hours sitting in front of a computer, chair yoga is a great way to stretch and relax your body, especially since you only need chair and comfortable clothes. This form of yoga is especially suitable for people withlimited mobility or physical disabilities because the chair offers extra support. What are you waiting for? Put on comfortable clothes, grab a chair and try this simple yoga sequence on the chair.

Step 1 - Sit on the edge of the chair

Sit on the edge of the chair with your back straight and place your hands on your waist. Take a few deep breaths.

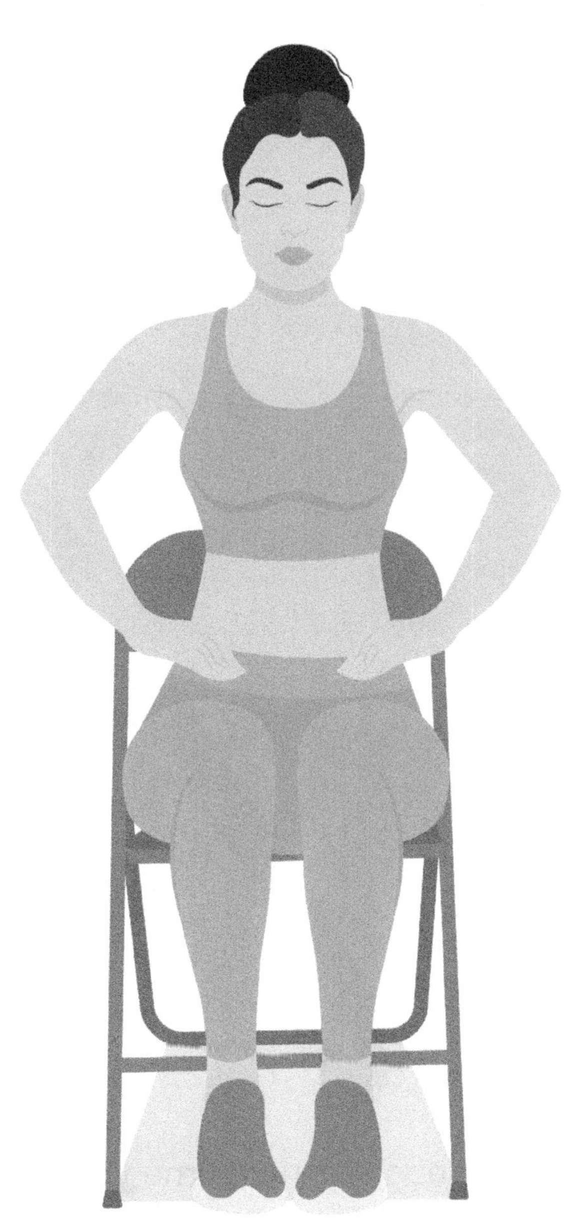

Step 2 - Cat-cow

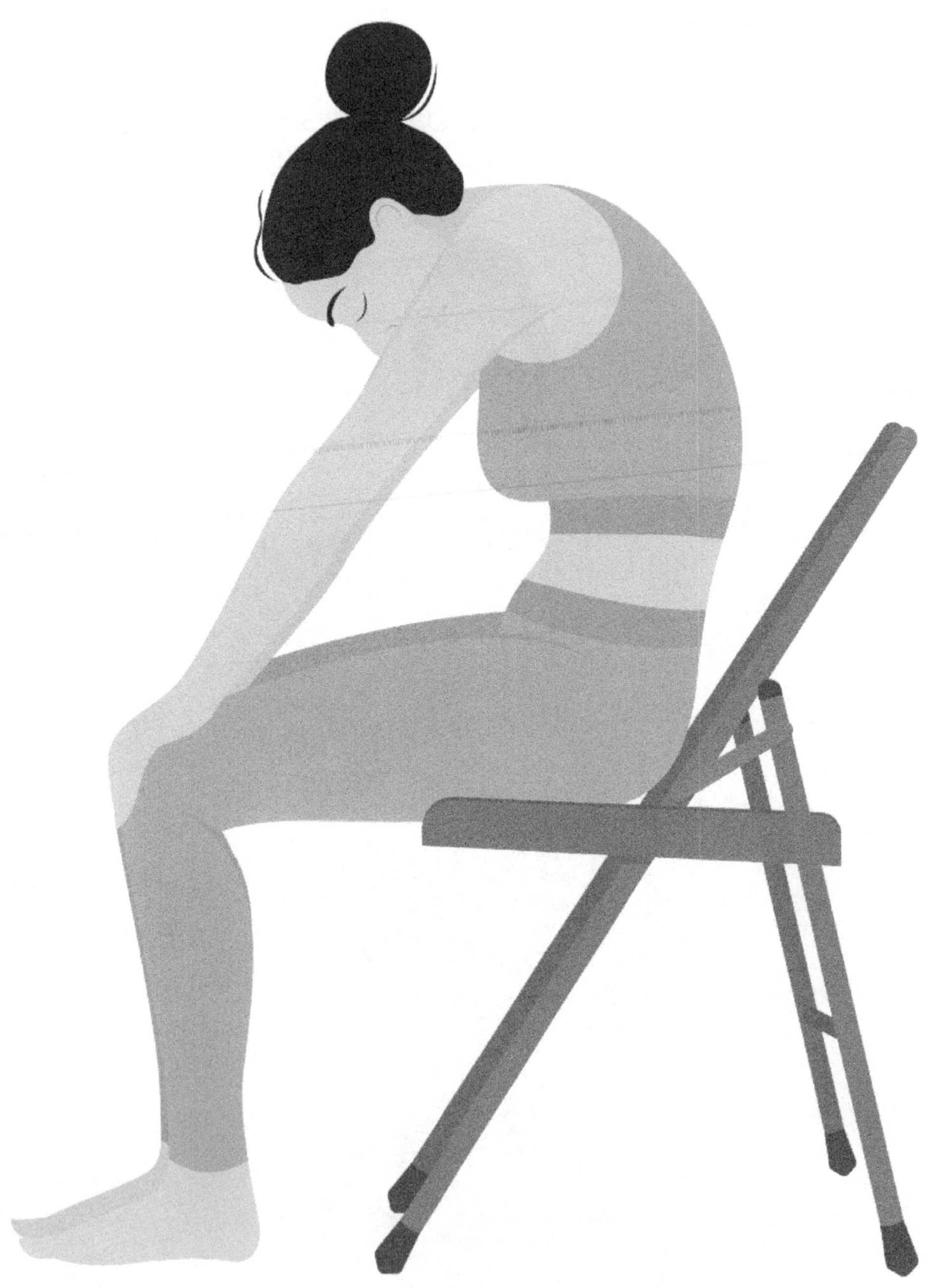

Put your hands on your knees and next time you inhale, arch yourback and look at the ceiling (cow). As you exhale, pull your abs inand curve your back (cat). Repeat this movement 5 times, following your breath, to relieve tension in the back and neck.

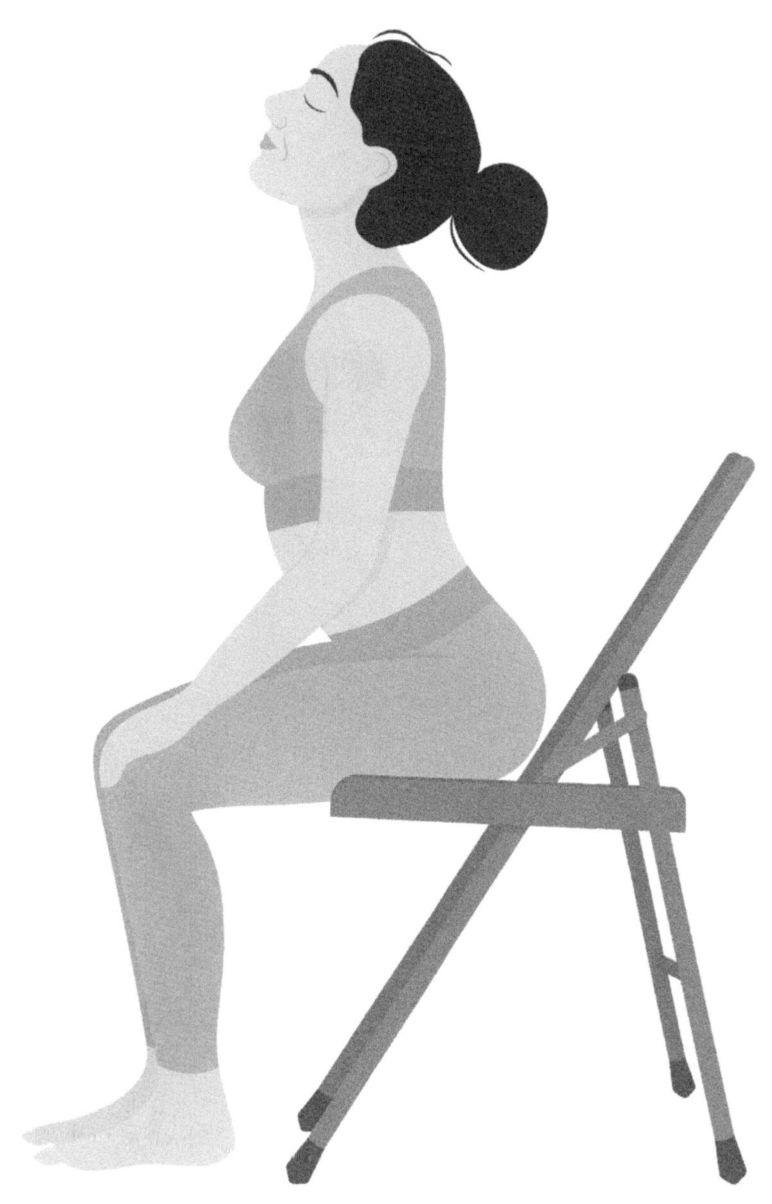

Step 3 – Urdhva Hastasana

Return to neutral position, lengthening the spine. The next time you inhale, raiseyour arms towards the ceiling. Stay in this position for a few seconds before lowering your arms as you exhale. Repeat this movement 5 times.

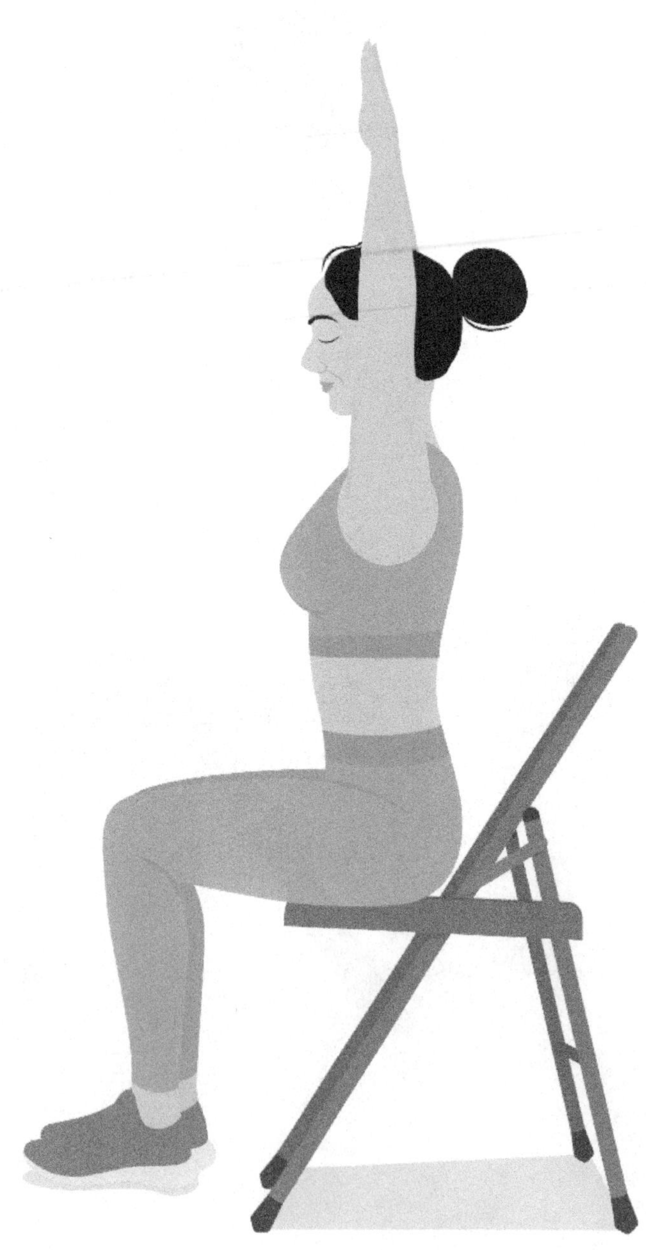

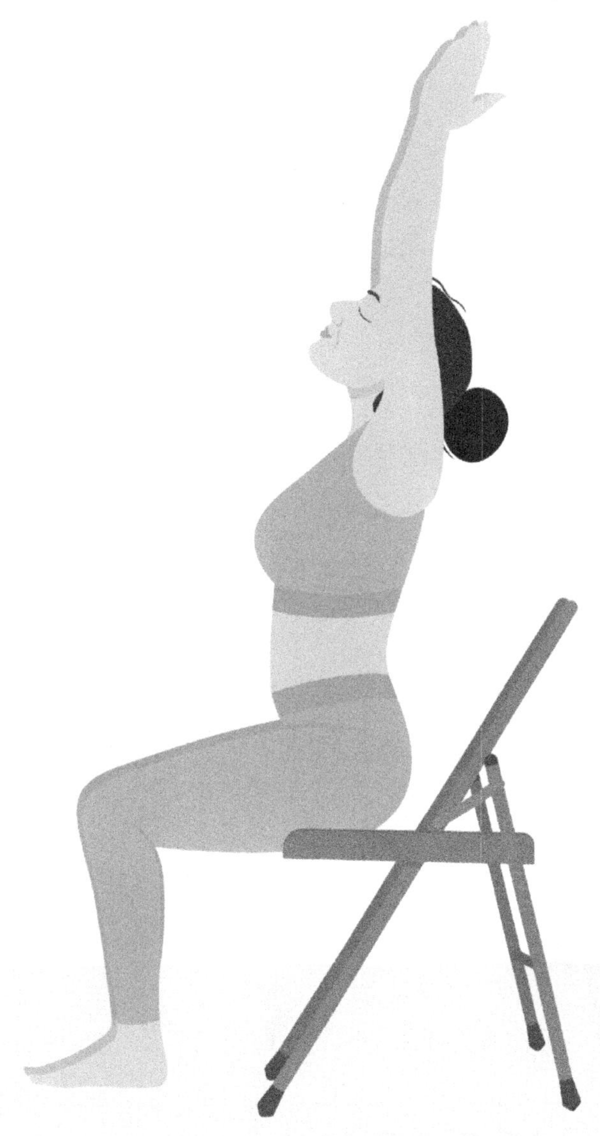

Step 4 - Sun Salutation

On the next inhalation, raise your arms again, this time pressing your palms together. Look towards the ceiling. On the next exhalation, let your arms float alongside your body. Repeat this movement 5 times.

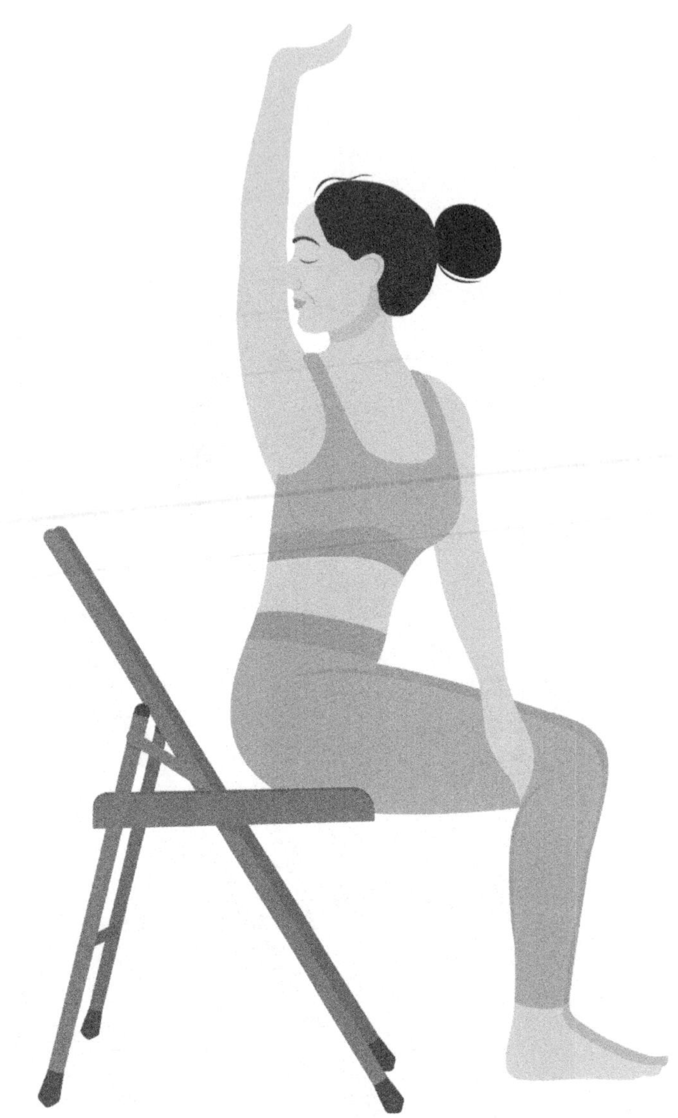

Step 5 - Back twist

On the next inhalation, raise your arms again, then turn right, placing your left hand against your right thigh and grasping the back of the chair with your right hand. As you exhale, return to center, raising your arms again, then turn left, placing your right hand against your left thigh and grasping the back of the chair with your left hand. Repeat 5 times on each side. When you are done, lower your arms.

Step 6 - Neck stretch

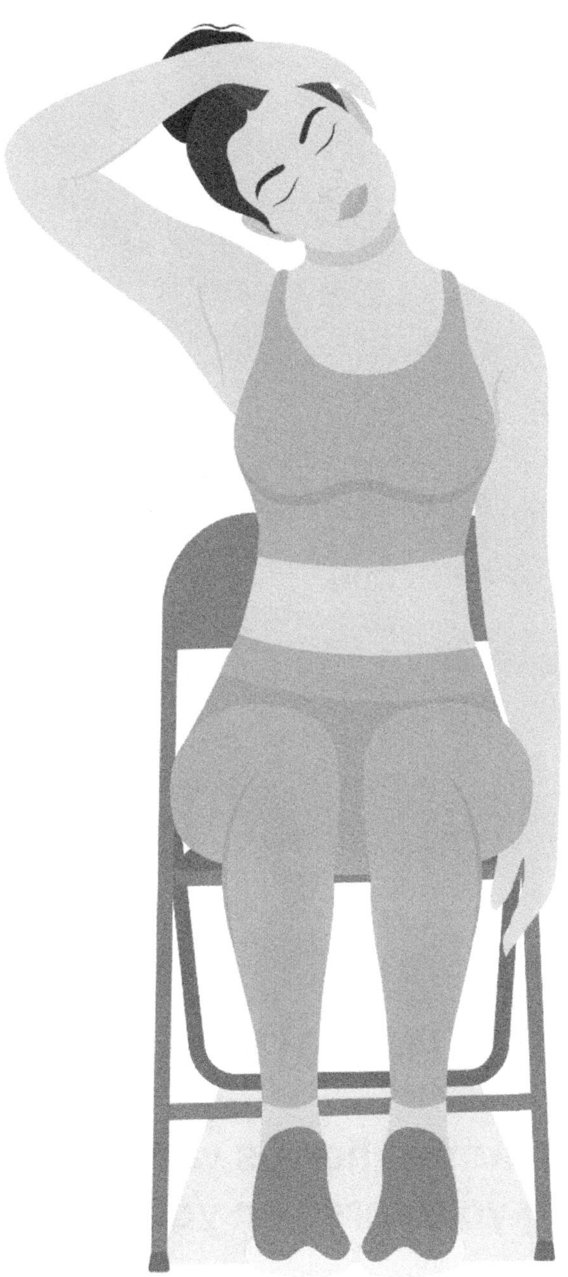

Bring your left hand to the left side of the chair, bring your right hand over your left ear and apply gentle pressure to stretch your neck. Count to 5 breaths, then repeat on the opposite side. At this point, interlace your fingers behind your head and apply gentle pressure to bring your chin towards your chest and stretch the back of your neck.

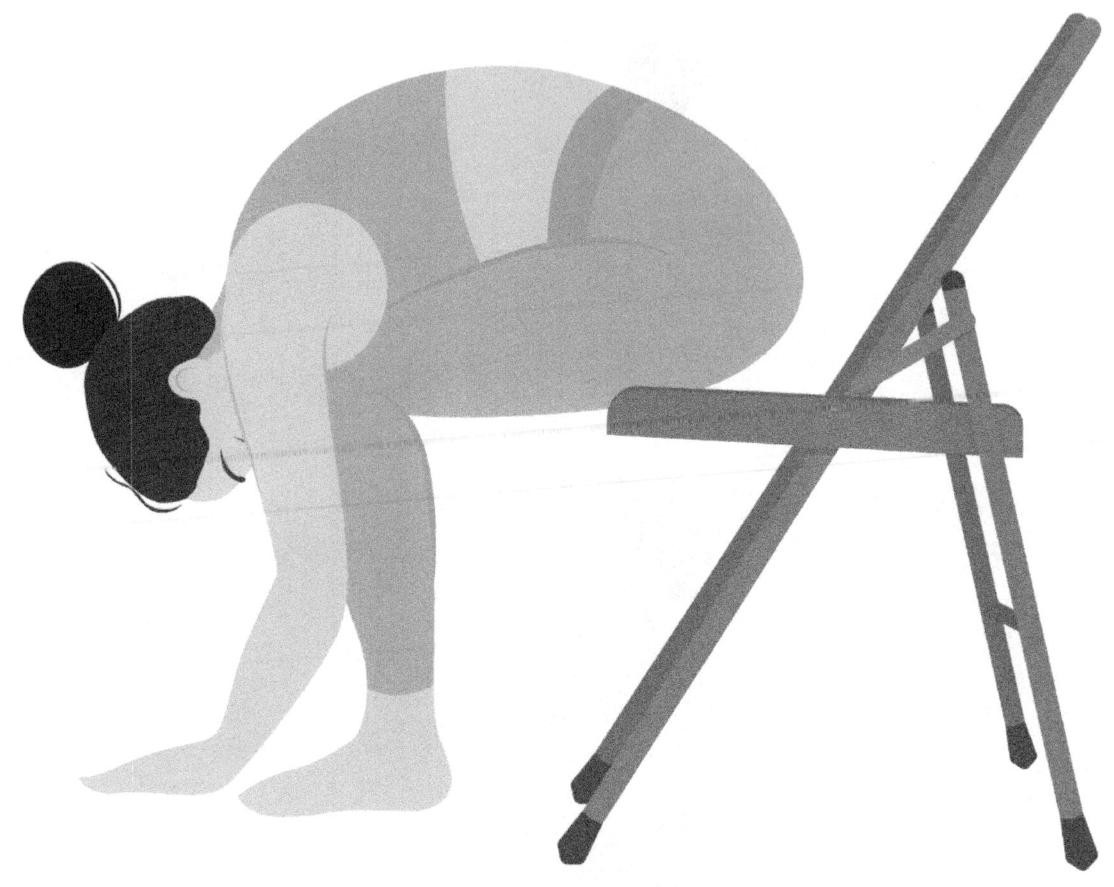

Step 7 – Uttanasana

Inhale and raise your arms, then as you exhale, lean forward, resting your torso on your thighs.

If possible, place your hands on the floor and dangle your head. Rest in this position for a few breaths. To finish, straighten your arms in front of you above your head and come up. Repeat three times in total and the last time you lean forward, stay there.

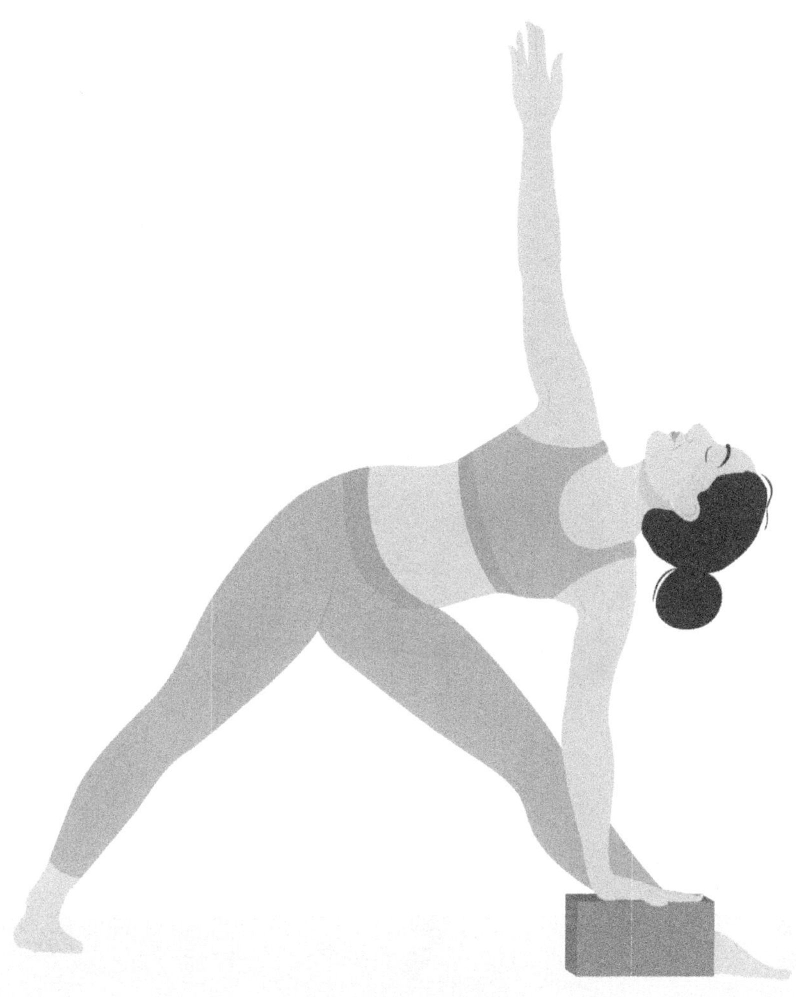

Step 8 – Utthita Parsvakonasana

Bring your left hand between your feet. Inhale and open the chest by rotating to the right, lifting the right arm upwards. Look towards the ceiling. Remain in this position for several breaths before lowering your right arm as you exhale. Repeat on the other side. If you have a hard time reaching the floor with your hand, you can use a block (or thick book) to get more height.

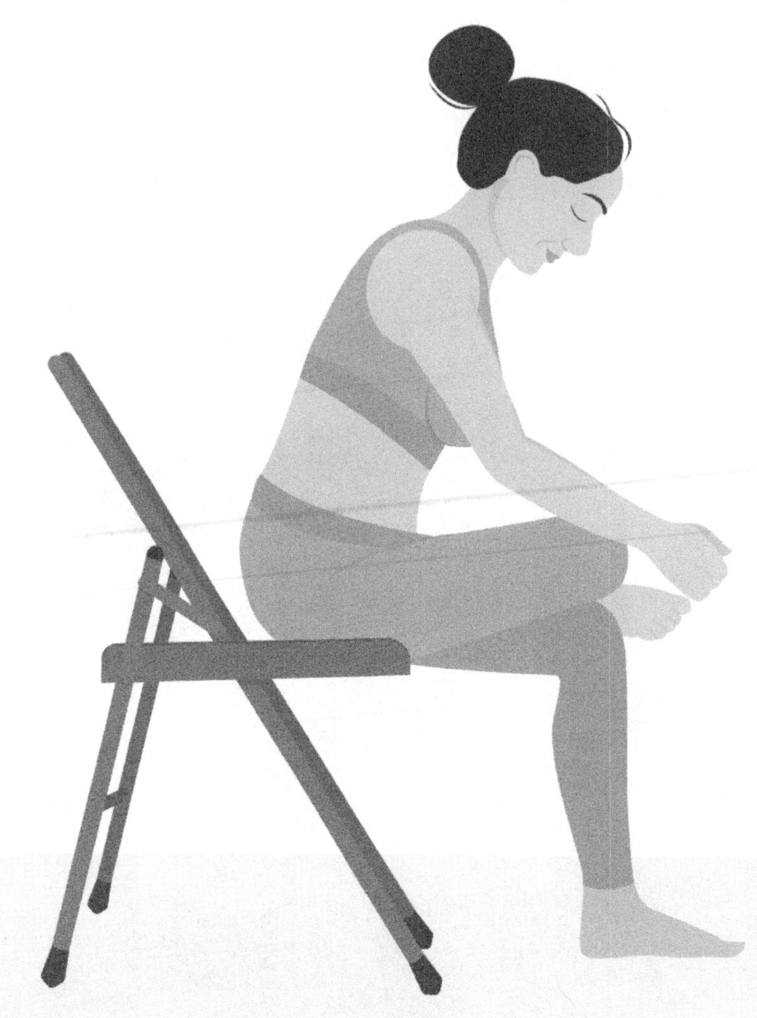

Step 9 - Eka Pada Rajakapotasana

Go back to your seat. Now, lift your right leg and bring your right ankle onto yourleft thigh, trying to keep the knee in line with the ankle as much as possible. If you want to increase the intensity, place your arms on your right leg and apply pressure to lower the knee further. Stay in this position for a few breaths beforerepeating with the other leg.

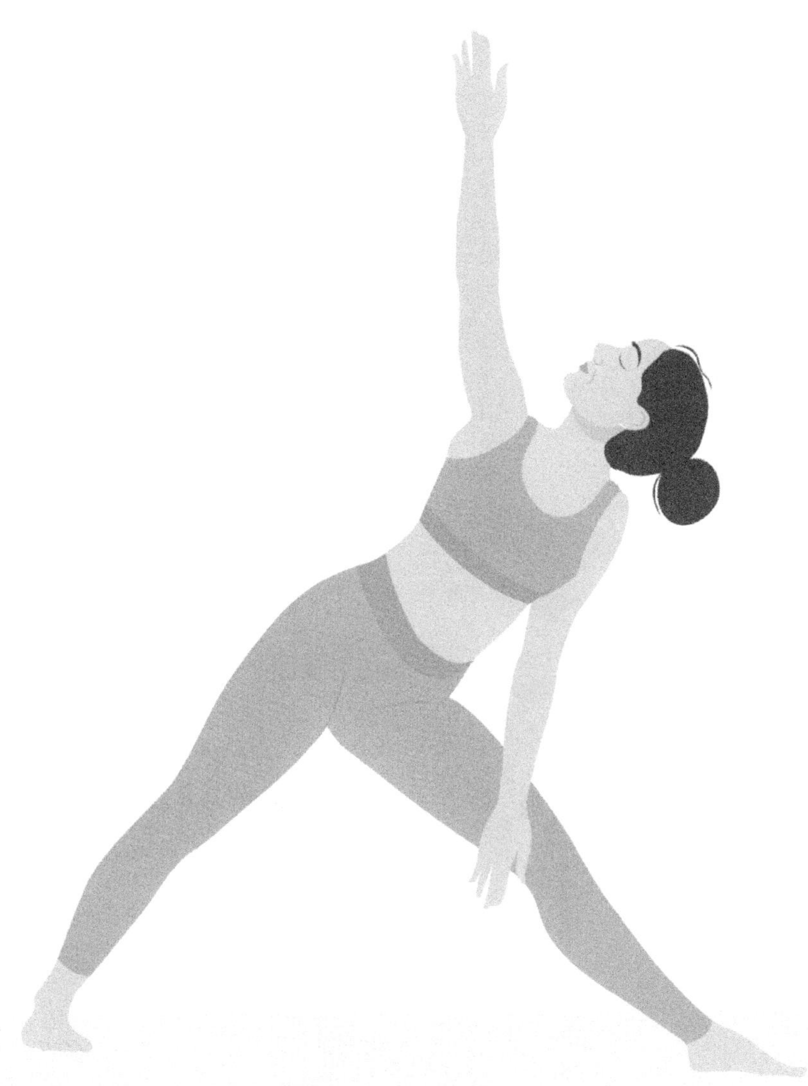

Step 10 - Opening the hips and twisting

Spread your legs and point your toes outward. Place your right arm against the inside of your right thigh, moving down to the floor. Raise your left arm towards the ceiling and look towards the left hand. Hold for five breaths, then repeat on the other side.

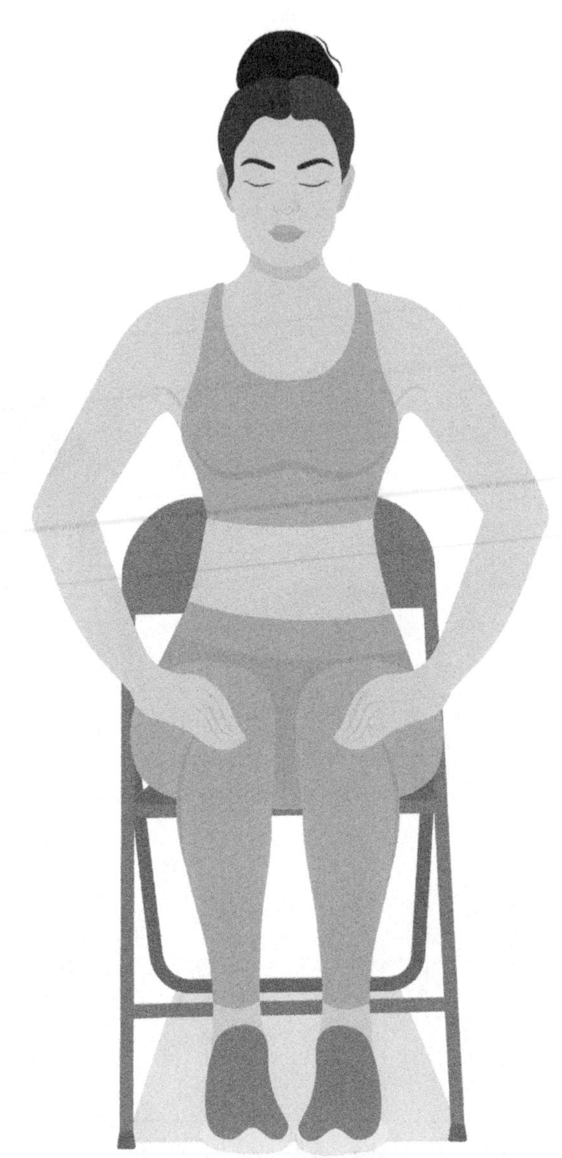

Step 11 – Savasana

Return to a sitting position with your back straight but relaxed. Place your handson your knees and close your eyes. Take a moment to relax and let your body absorb the benefits of this practice. When you are ready, open your eyes again.

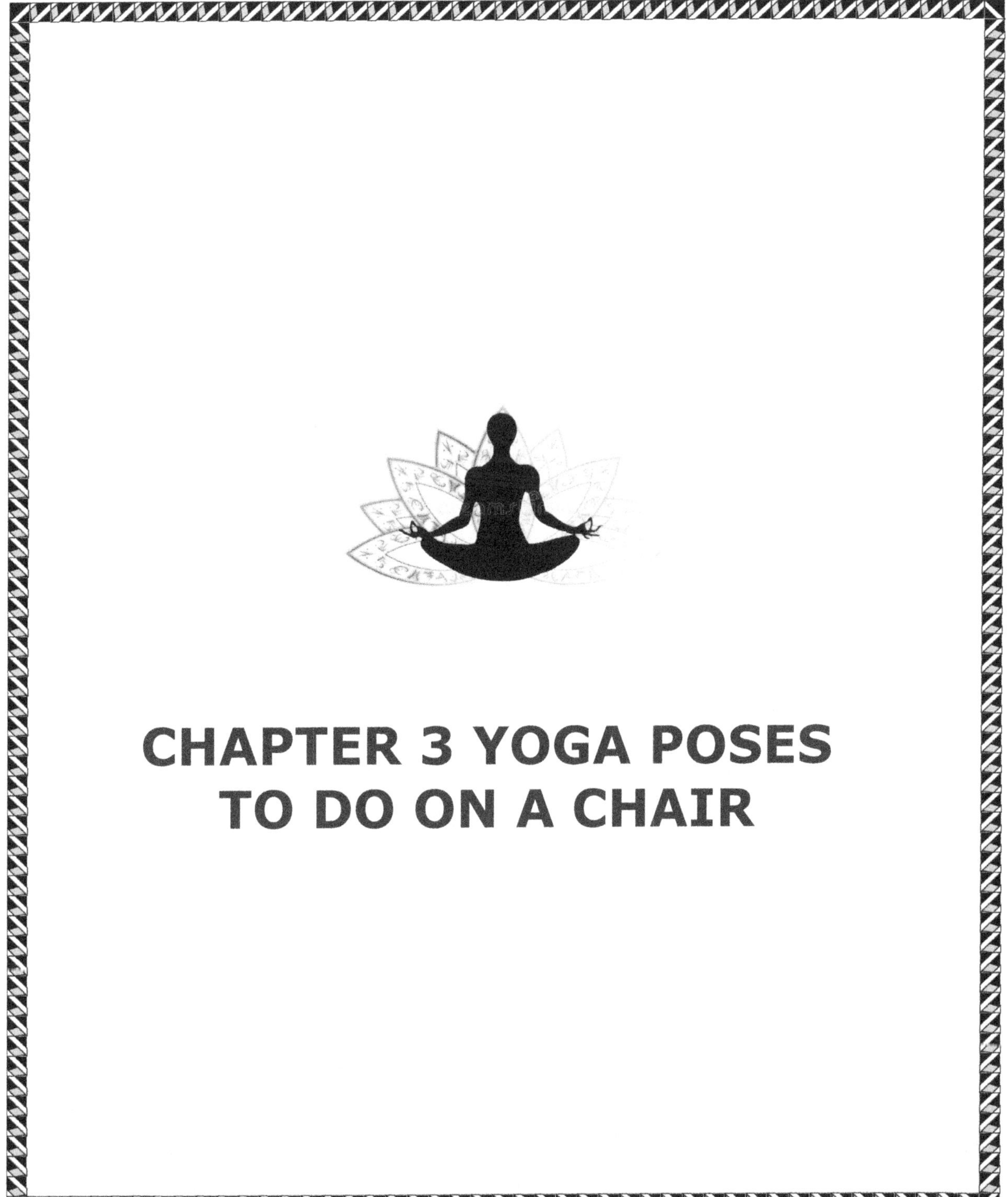

CHAPTER 3 YOGA POSES TO DO ON A CHAIR

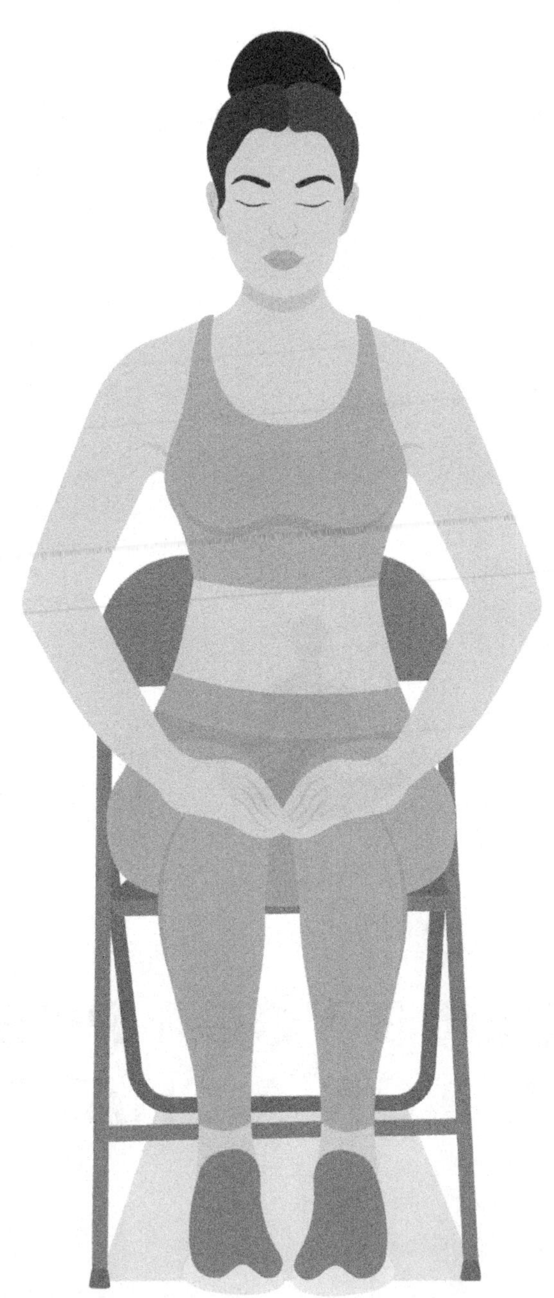

Breathing practice

For your breathing practice, sit on the chair with your back straight and rest yourfeet firmly on the floor.

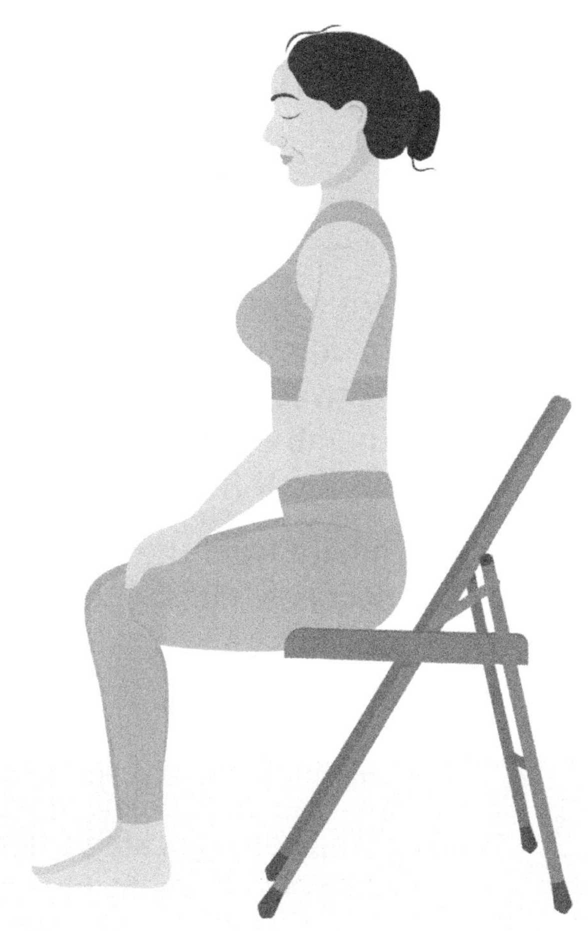

Box Breath

Close your eyes and place your hands on your thighs;

Inhale with diaphragmatic breathing for 4 seconds;

Hold your breath for 4 seconds;

Exhale through your mouth for 4 seconds;

Pause for 4 seconds;

Inhale again recreating the whole sequence at least 5-6 times.

Alternating nostril breathing

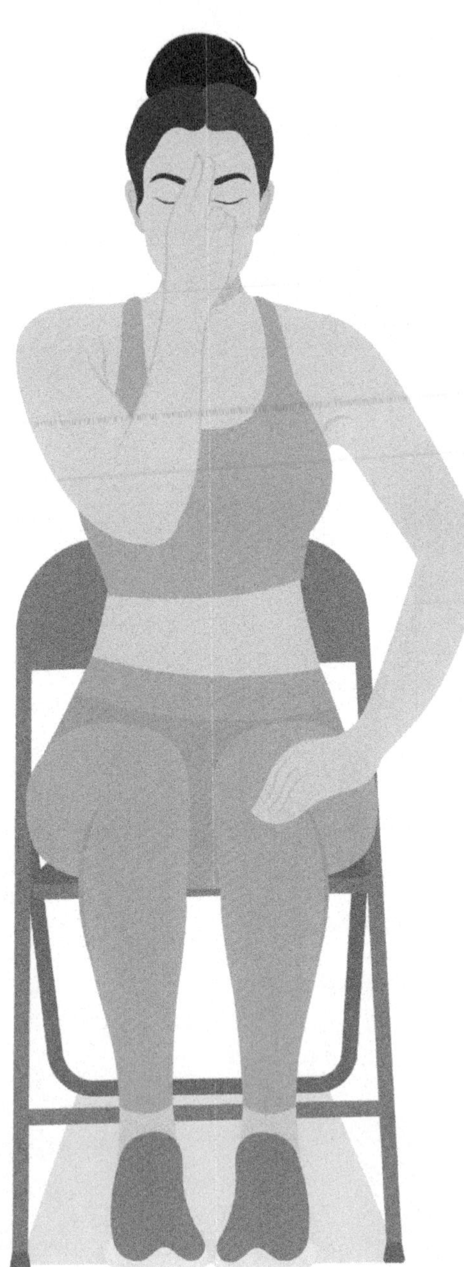

Place your left hand on your thigh;

With the right hand, place the index and middle fingers on the forehead, in thespace between the two eyebrows and place the thumb on the right nostril and the ring finger on the left nostril;

Inhale from the right nostril for a few seconds, closing the left nostril with the ring finger;

Hold the breath for 4 seconds

and then, blocking the right nostril with the thumb, exhale from the left nostrilthat you left free from the ring finger;

Do the reverse procedure:

inhale from the left nostril blocking the right, hold for a few seconds and then exhale from the right nostril blocking the left;

Go on alternating your breathing for a few minutes.

Torsion of the vertebral column

Sit comfortably in the chair, placing your feet firmly on the ground;

Take a deep inhalation;

As you exhale, gently rotate your torso to the right by turning your head as well, placing your left hand on your right knee and your right hand on the back of the chair;
Hold the twist for 3-4 breaths and then gently return to the starting position;

At this point do your twist on the left side: inhale and then exhale gently rotate your torso and head to the left, placing your right hand on your left knee and your left hand on the back of thechair;

Hold this position for 3-4 breaths and then return to the starting position; Proceed, alternating the 2 rotations for at least 2-3 minutes.

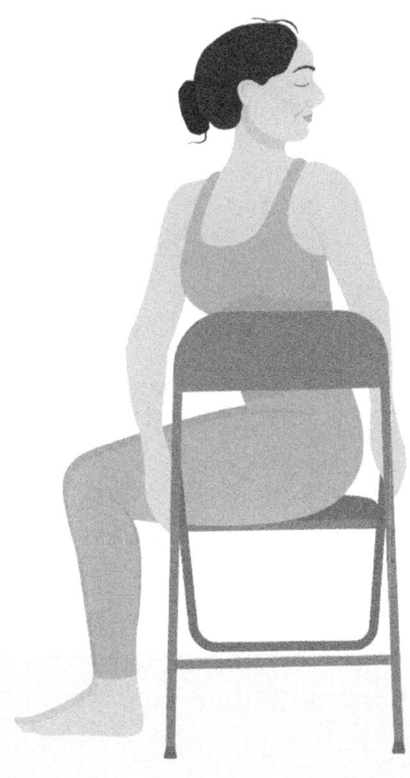

Stretching for the ankles

Among the seated yoga positions, we can do some simple stretching exercises to stretch the muscles.

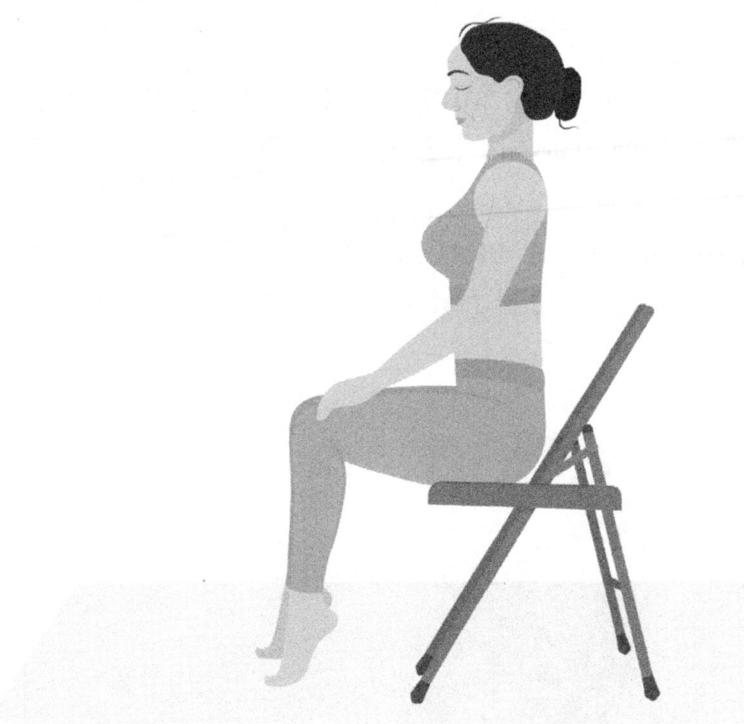

Heel lift

Get comfortable in the chair with your back straight and leaned back;

Put your feet on the floor and if the chair is too high, help yourself with yoga supports;

Place your hands on

your thighs; As you

inhale through your nose,

point your toes on the floor (or blocks)and lift your heels as high as possible;

Exhale and lower your heels;

Repeat the sequence for at least ten breaths.

Circles with the ankle

Sit well with your back straightand resting on the backrest and your feet firmly on the ground;

Raise your right leg, without exaggerating and begin to rotate your ankle clockwise for at least 5 times,stop and make another 5 rotations counterclockwise;

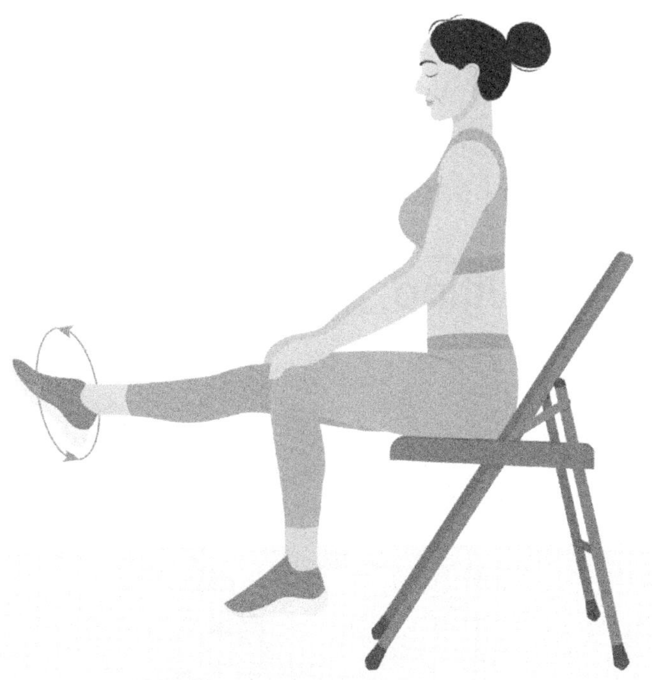

Put your feet back on the ground and lift your left leg,

repeating the rotation with the left ankle first in one direction and then in theother;

Return the leg to the starting position and take a few breaths to rest;

When you feel ready, lift your right leg and resume the rotations of theankle, and then switch to the other leg.

Do this at least 3 times per leg.

Rag doll yoga position

This position is called the rag doll because you will stretch andrelax your neck, shoulders and back going to bend forward, inthe classic position of the rag doll.

Here's how to do it.

As a starting position this time,

we sit with the back straight and the legs slightly apart,a little wider than the hips; At this point lean forward little by little, letting yourself fall and relaxing your shoulders,head and arms that you will let dangle;

Bend as much as you can but without forcing the position,

and in the meantime, continue to inhale and exhale deeply;

Hold the position for a few breaths and then slowly begin to rise with the back vertebra after vertebra, leaving the head for last;

Take a few breaths while sitting, and then repeat.

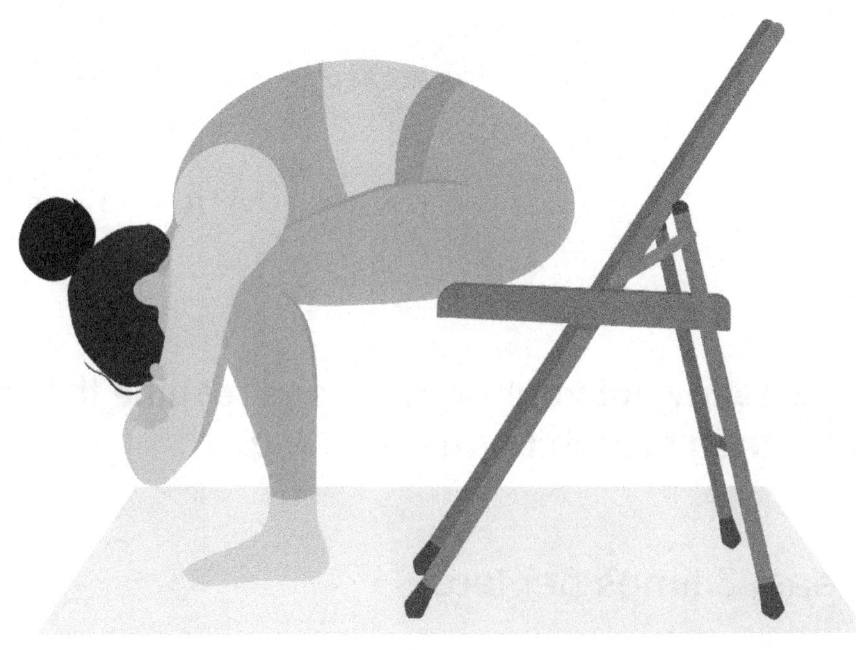

CHAPTER 4 EXERCISES TO DO IN THE OFFICE

Yoga is a discipline suitable for everyone, that's for sure!

But for those in a sedentary job, the benefits of the practice are even more.

People often joke that “this job destroys me!”

Actually, it could be true.

Stress is the main culprit when it comes to occupational health, but there

is another danger lurking in the office: a sedentary lifestyle.

According to Wired magazine "Sitting is the new smoking". Scientific evidence correlates a highly sedentary lifestyle to a shorter life span.

Sedentary people have an increased risk of developing heart disease, cancer anddiabetes. Added to this are the pain and muscle tension often caused by poor posture.

Anyone who spends more than eight hours a day sitting is at risk, even if they exercise regularly.

Hunching over your desk often leads to a weakening of the abdominal area and leads to imbalances in the neck, upper back and chest muscles.

Due to our collective reliance on keyboards, screens and smartphones, we are becoming a generation with hunched shoulders and necks.

Of course, most of us can't just leave office work for a healthier alternative.

So, what can we do about it?

We can do some desk yoga. . . at the office!

The **main cause** of health problems is impaired blood circulation in the pelvic region.

The **deterioration of blood circulation** in the legs often leads to varicose veins.

The compression and lack of blood circulation in the abdominal region deal a severe blow to the digestive system. Hence constant constipation, indigestion, gas, heartburn, sleepiness and other problems.

Sitting for a long time in one position causes severe fatigue, and also contributes to the development of a variety of diseases (hemorrhoids, osteochondrosis, radiculitis, prostatitis, etc.).

A **sedentary lifestyle** contributes to the curvature of the spine. Even correct posture cannot always prevent compression of the lumbar vertebrae.

Another consequence of a sedentary lifestyle is shallow breathing, which makes things worse in general.

To cope with the negative consequences of a sedentary lifestyle, you need to find a way to increase flexibility and mobility - in other words, you need to movemore!

Instead of having another coffee, do some asanas!

Yoga helps relax muscles, relieve pain, energize and take your mind off work.

A good rule of thumb is 50/10.

For every 50 minutes of working, dedicate 10 minutes to movement. Breaking away from sitting hours with just a few minutes of movement can reduce all those risk factors and make you feel focused, rested and healthy.

Regular yoga practice can help offset the damage caused by sitting all day.

If you are a yoga beginner, I propose 8 positions to do directly in the office to reduce muscle tension, reduce stress and calm the mind.

You don't have to change your clothes or roll out a mat and run a full sequence;just think about moving a bit!

Take a little walk in the office (or outside if you can get away from it), take the stairs instead of the elevator, and do yoga at your desk!

Doing yoga at your desk is a great way to move and stretch your body muscles without having to distract colleagues or leave the office.

The best part about desk yoga is that it takes very little time, you can do it discreetly with your office outfit.

8 DESK YOGA POSES YOU CAN PRACTICE DURING YOUR WORKDAY

There are many yoga positions that you can do even while you are sitting at yourdesk, they are variations of the classic yoga asanas, designed specifically to be performed in a sitting position, in a discreet way, even when we are in public and we do not want to distract people.

The seated twist

This pose is a great way to start your "office yoga" session.

Keep your feet parallel on the floor.

Place your right hand on the left armrest (or seat) of the chair,keep your back straight and look over your left shoulder.

With each inhalation, stretch your back, breathing deeply.

With each exhalation, deepen the twist (but without going beyond your limit).Hold for a few breaths, then repeat on the opposite side.

This position will help you reset your posture and will immediately relieve you of major tensions! it's a handy way to move a little bit.

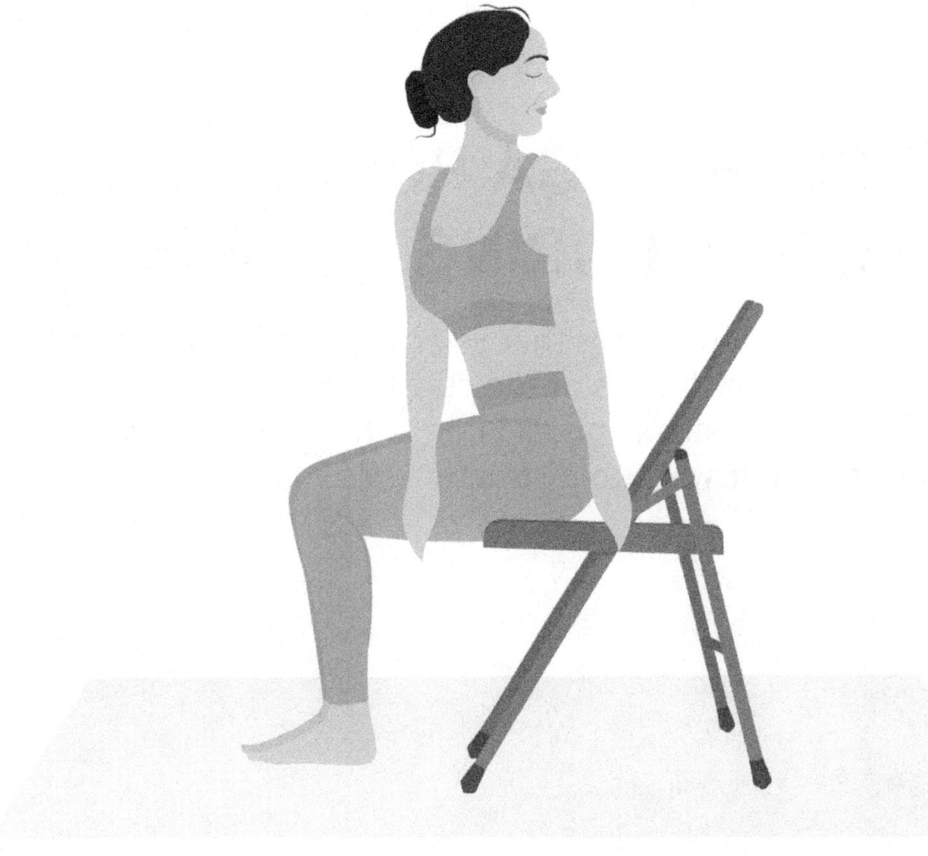

Mountain position at work

This pose is a great way to introduce some yoga into your day. Whether you areat your desk, in your study or even in the coffee area, no one will notice that you are actually doing yoga!

Keep the soles of your feet firmly on the ground and relax your hands at your sides, try to slowly straighten your back, with the top of your head reaching towards the sky. Close your eyes if you feel comfortable and focus on your breath.

Hold the position for as many breaths as you like (also depending on the time you have available). Allow yourself to become aware of your body and breath - it's a great way to create peace in your busy workday and also bring more awareness to your posture. Don't you want to get up from your chair?

Stay seated and open your knees by spreading them wider than your hips. From there, lean your torso forward towards the floor. At this point your hands may touch the ground, depending on your flexibility. It is important not to force things. Whichever variation you choose, let your head dangle and feel its weight as it helps you stretch your muscles and releases tension in your head and neck. Enjoy the fresh blood flow to the brain - you will feel energized and refreshed after staying in this position for several breaths.

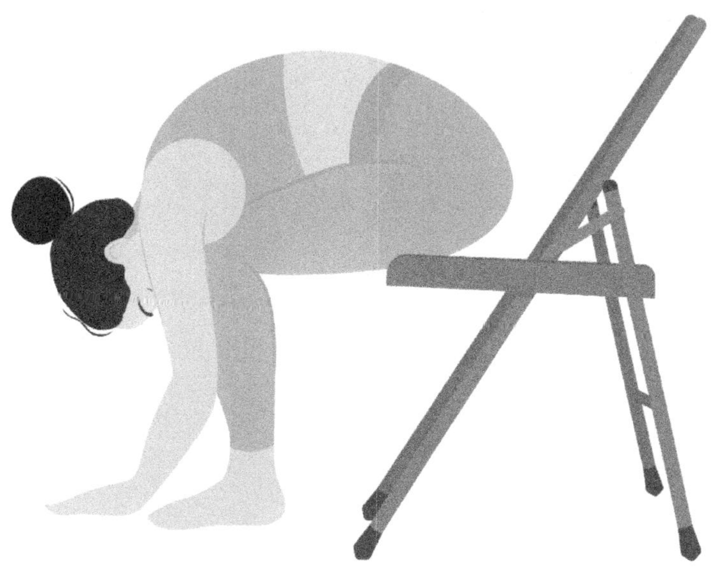

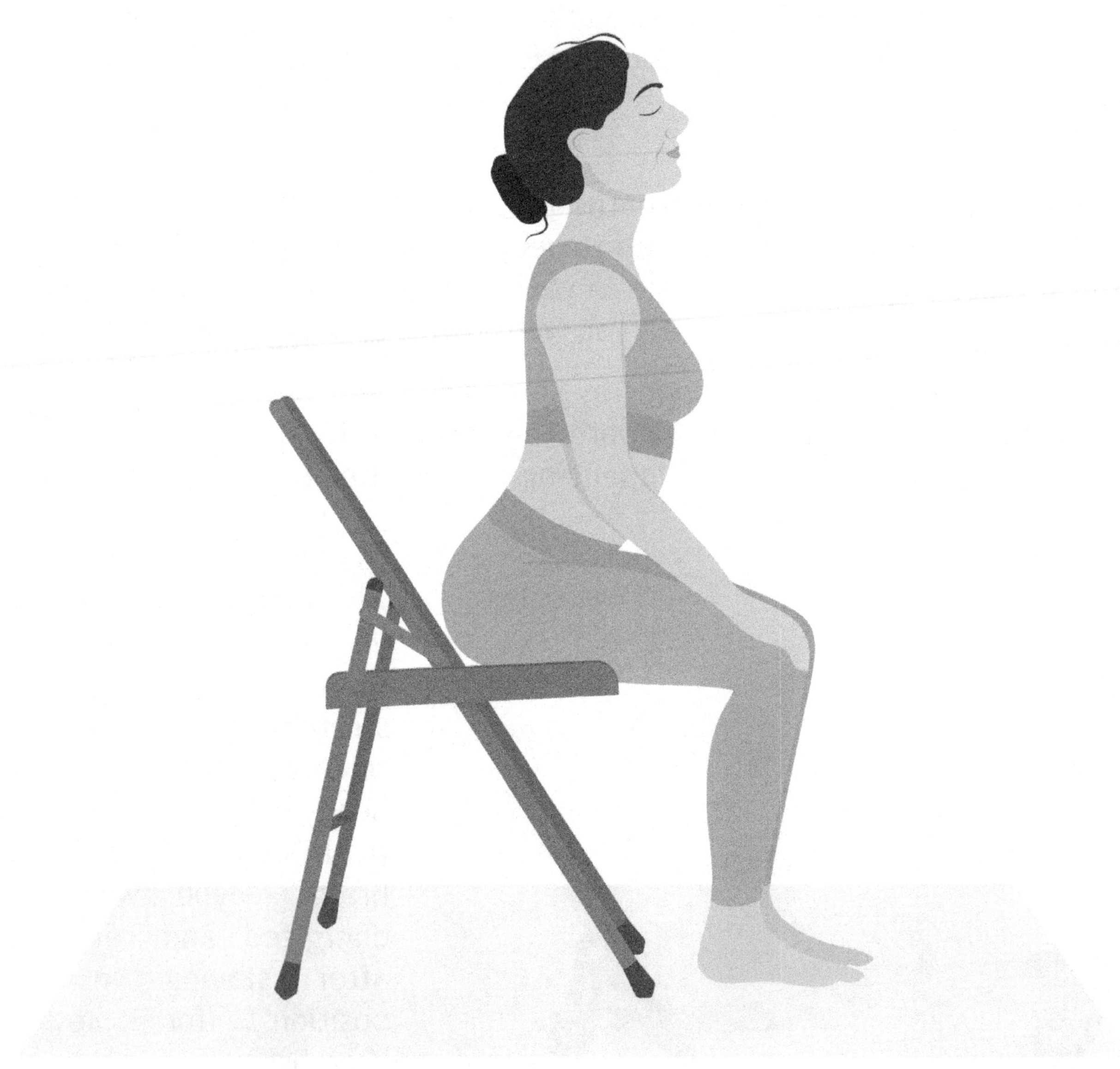

Eagle stance

The eagle position that I propose is a variation that can be performed while seated to stretch the upper back and shoulders.

Extend your arms parallel in front of you.

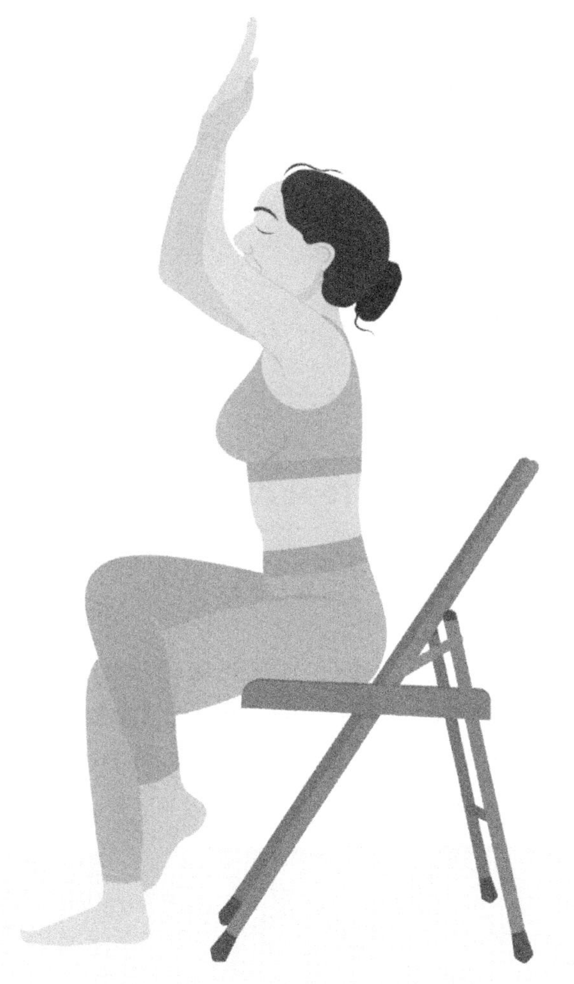

Cross them, making sure your right arm is over your left.Now fold your arms and raise your forearms up, bringing them perpendicular to the floor, continue the intertwining of the hands until you get to join the palms.

If you can't, you can stay in the previous step and press the backs of your handsagainst each other.

Don't let the chest close, rather keep it open. The shoulder blades should remain down. Hold the position by breathing deeply for up to a minute or as long as you can. But try to increase the time each time you do it.

At this point, gently release the position and perform it on the other side.

Half lotus at the desk

Sitting on the chair, gently place your left ankle in the crease of your right hip.

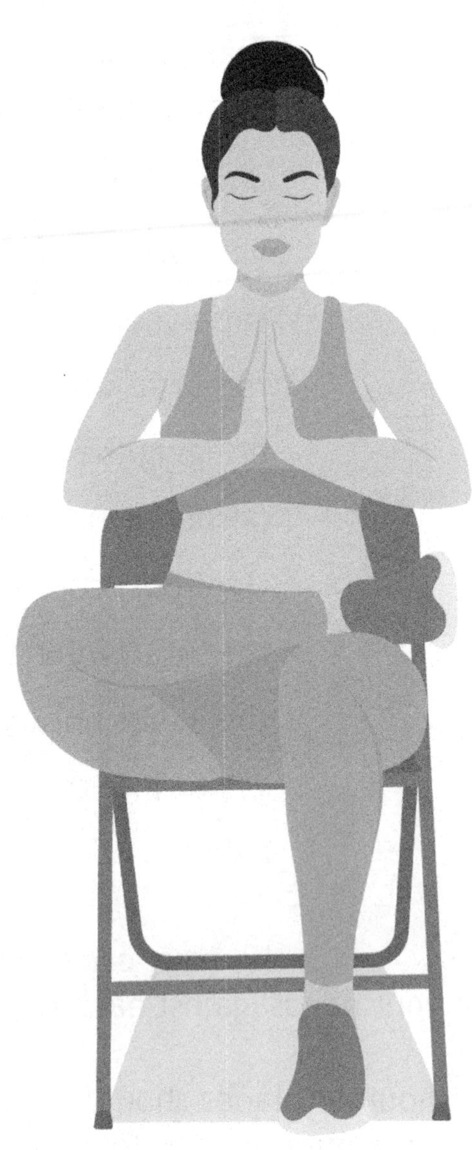

This movement requires a fairly deep hip opening, so work onit gradually.

Keep your left foot flexed and relax your left knee.

If this is too intense for you, simply relax the lower left foot on the inside of theright thigh.

Stay here for five deep breaths and then switch sides.

This hip opening is a great way to counter the tension that builds up in the hipjoint after long periods of sitting time - the perfect desk yoga pose!

Full yoga lotus position

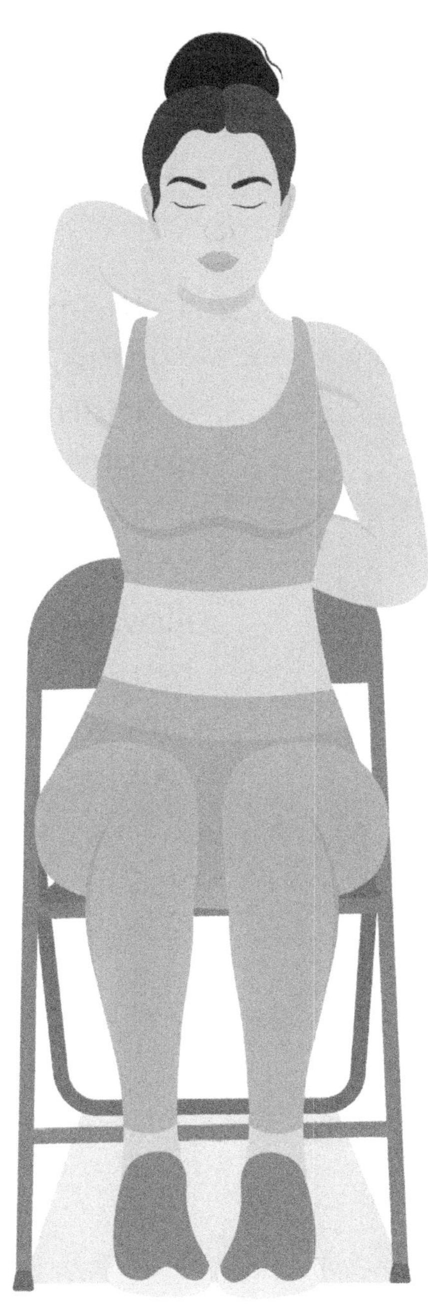

Traditionally, this pose includes moving the legs as well,but right now we focus on the upper body.

Sit upright with your buttocks resting on the chair evenly, trying to stay comfortable. Raise your right hand by extending your arm, then bend your elbow bringing your hand behind your neck.

At this point the left hand behind the back, in the center of the dorsal area. Try joining your hands to feel the stretch in the triceps.

If your shoulders are particularly stiff, use a strap or towel between your hands to help you get into the position

Hold for 3-5 breaths, then switch sides.

Sitting Crescent Moon

Start by raising your arms above your head,join your palms by crossing your fingers and straighten the index fingers of both hands.As you exhale, bend over to one side, creating a crescent shape with your body.

For a fuller expression of the pose, twist your chest to the sky and look up.Hold the side bend for 2-3 deep breaths, then repeat on the other side.

The crescent moon yoga position deeply stretches the hips and spine, also improves circulation and promotes concentration, allowing you to return to your work with better awareness.

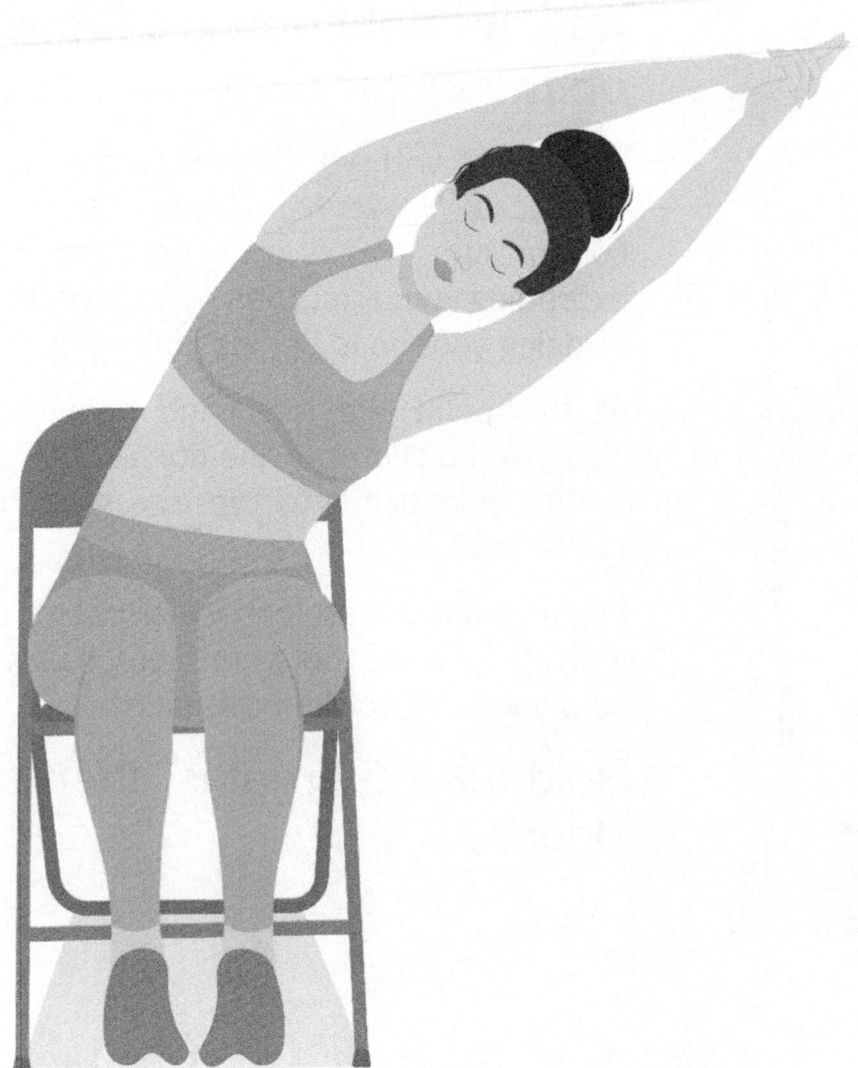

The "domestic pigeon"

This is a variant of the more classic royal pigeon, to be performed seated at the desk with the help of a chair.

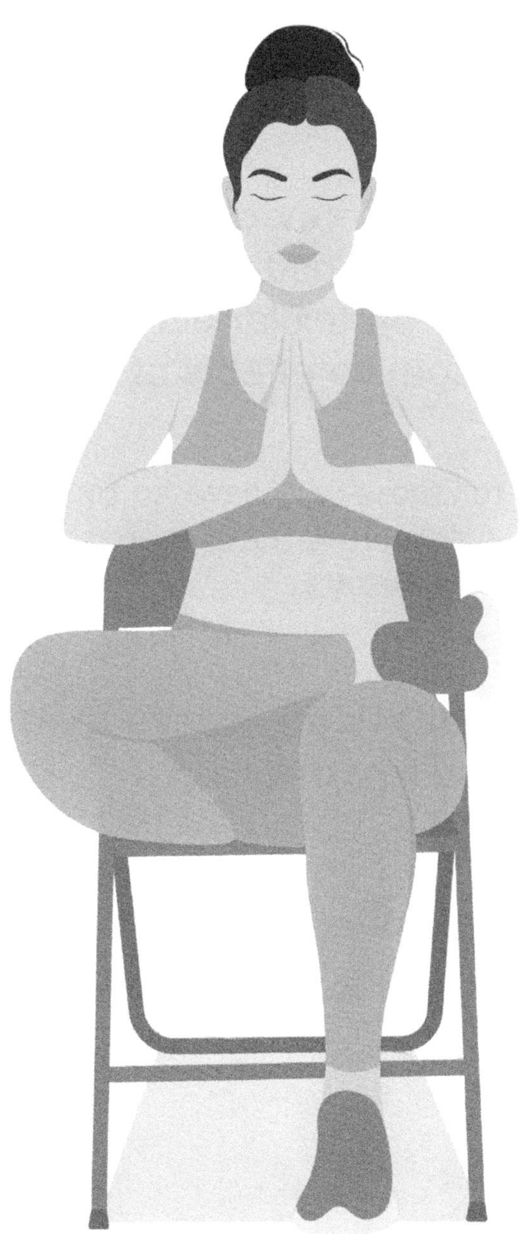

While sitting, place one leg over the other by placing the ankle above the knee, forming a 90-degree angle.
Flex your foot so you don't put pressure on the knee.Maintaining the erect position, with the weight of the body well distributed on the ischium,slowly lean forward

until you begin to feel a moderate stretch of the lateral band of the thigh, holding the position for 5-10 breaths.

Then repeat on the other side.

Desk yoga can make a difference to your body and mind

Not only does regular yoga practice provide immediate relief to tense and aching muscles, it also strengthens the core by improving posture. Abdominal muscles in particular play a vital role in improving back pain and other negative effects of sitting for a long time.

It is a way to train and burn calories even for those who have no time and for those who are too lazy to go to the gym. Incorporate these exercises into your work routine and you will soon discover the results.

Incorporating desk yoga into your workday is an excellent way to bring your yoga practice to work.

Your body and mind will thank you for it.

Be kind to yourself, hold each asana for 5-6 breaths and then move on to the next, keeping your attention on the breath!

CHAPTER 5 EXAMPLES OF ADVANCED CHAIR YOGA TRAINING

When I did my first yoga class on the chair, I did not think it would be so successful.

Instead, there are many people who for various reasons cannot practice yoga onthe mat but would like to do it.

For those who practice regularly, it seems impossible that there are some who are not able to stay even in Adho Mukha Svanasana, "downward-looking dog", but unfortunately it is true.

Many people who have been standing still for many years, overweight, with motorproblems, veterans of injuries, during pregnancy, or are frightened, or simply find themselves uncomfortable being in positions very different from the common daily movement.

The good news is that many have a great desire to move and get back in the game and get back in shape.

These are simple and safe exercises that anyone can do at home. However, if you are suffering from any pathology, it is always better to consult your doctor before doing any type of activity, even this one.

I also recommend that you use a stable chair, heavy enough to prevent you fromfalling to the ground.

Remember that the chair is a help, never a substitute for your body. Never entrust your Asana to the chair. It is you who must always have the situation under control.

Basic position

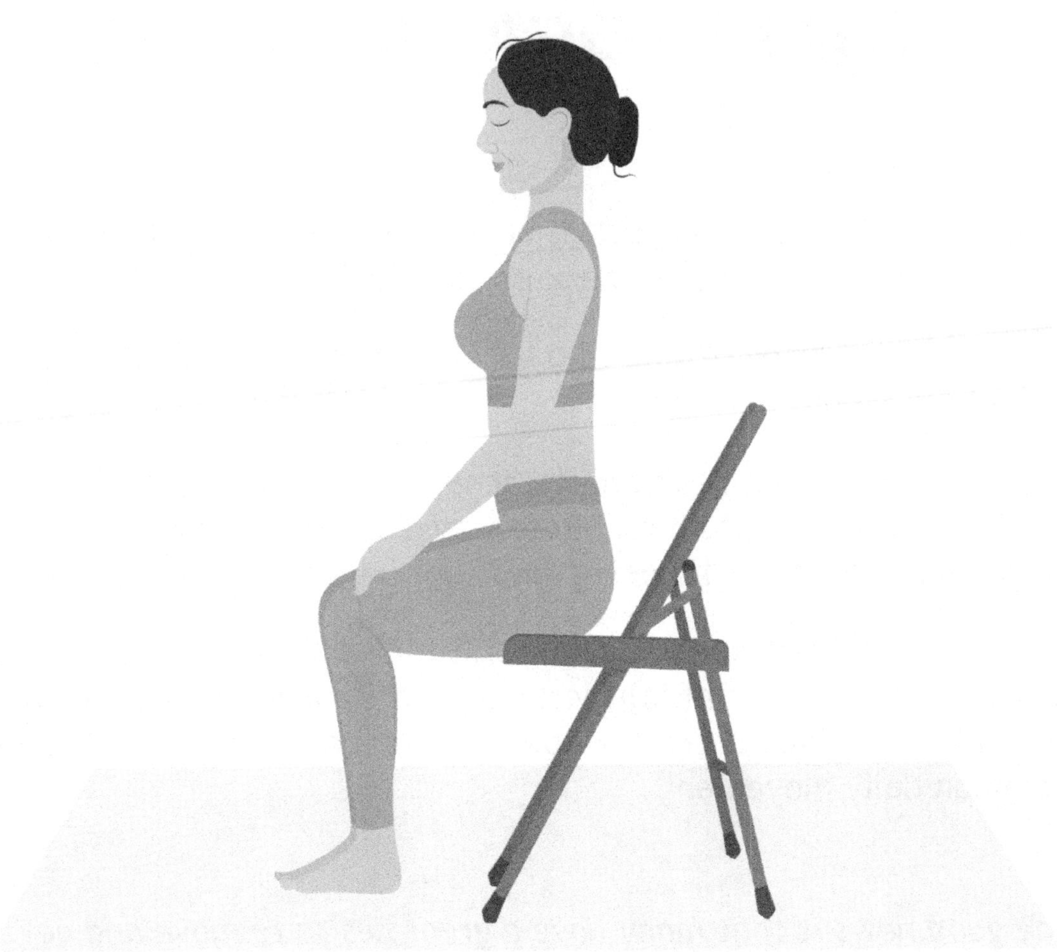

The basic position for doing this activity on the chair is sitting.

The buttocks rest on the seat but the back is detached from the backrest and well stretched.

The feet must be firmly placed on the ground. If you are of short stature, you may have to bring your seat to the front of the chair to have your feet supported or opt for a lower chair, or a stool. In any case, the feet must never be suspended.

The legs are not together, check that your feet and knees are aligned with the width of your hips.

Starting position: Seated Utthanasana

Utthanasana is a forward bend with the legs straight.

The seated version is very similar in principle but having the legs bent is much less invasive for the back, ideal if you have poor lumbar mobility.

From the basic sitting position, we inhale while stretching the back upwards and then exhaling we place our hands on the knees and slowly go down to bring the chest towards the thighs and the chin beyond the knees.

The legs remain aligned hips widthwise, avoid opening the knees sideways, and the feet always well supported.

Do not force the descent but stop in a position in which you feel comfortable butabove all do not lift your buttocks from the seat. When you feel that they beginto rise, stop.

Take 10 to 15 long diaphragmatic breaths in this position.

To rise, close your abdominals well, push the soles of your feet firmly to the ground and slowly unroll your back to bring it back to the starting position.

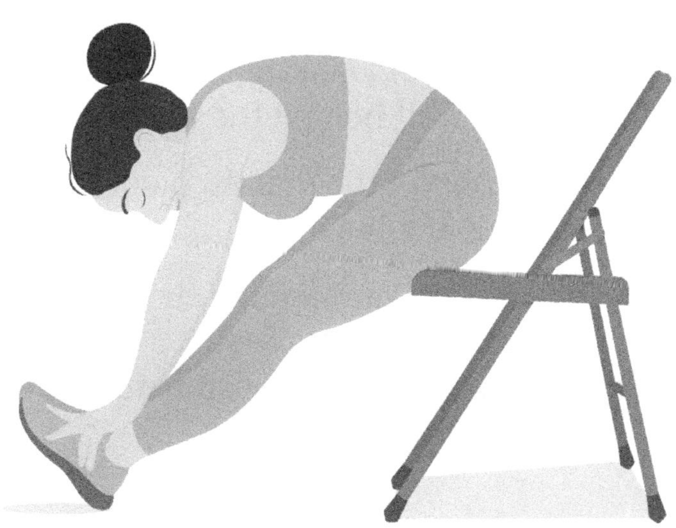

Seated Garudasana

The sacred eagle pose of yoga can also be performed while seated, even eagles often stay on their nests on mountain tops and this does not make them any less regal.

From the basic position we cross the right leg over the left and bring the left footto the center.

If it is possible for us, the toe of the right foot hooks under the left calf, if it is impossible, or to be able to do this we must take a position that does not allow us to remain seated in the basic position with the back straight and extended, let's be content to keep the foot near the calf.

We bring our left elbow in front of the shoulders at a 90-degree angle, keeping the shoulders relaxed.

The right arm, passing from underneath, twists onto the left arm which, however, must not lose the 90-degree angle. Ideally the right-hand rests palm topalm with the left hand, but if this is not possible, we remain in the position closest to this ideal.

Once in this position the back tends to stretch even more upward while the leftfoot pushes hard towards the floor, as if we wanted to get up by pushing only with one leg.

The elbows push in front of us as if wanting to move away from the body by spreading the shoulder blades well behind the back.

With the elbows always pushed, the hands point upwards, keeping the shoulderslow, pushing towards the buttocks.

The position, if done well is very demanding, try it for a few times before making it very intense and when you feel it, keep it for 10 - 15 long breaths and then do it again with the opposite side of the body.

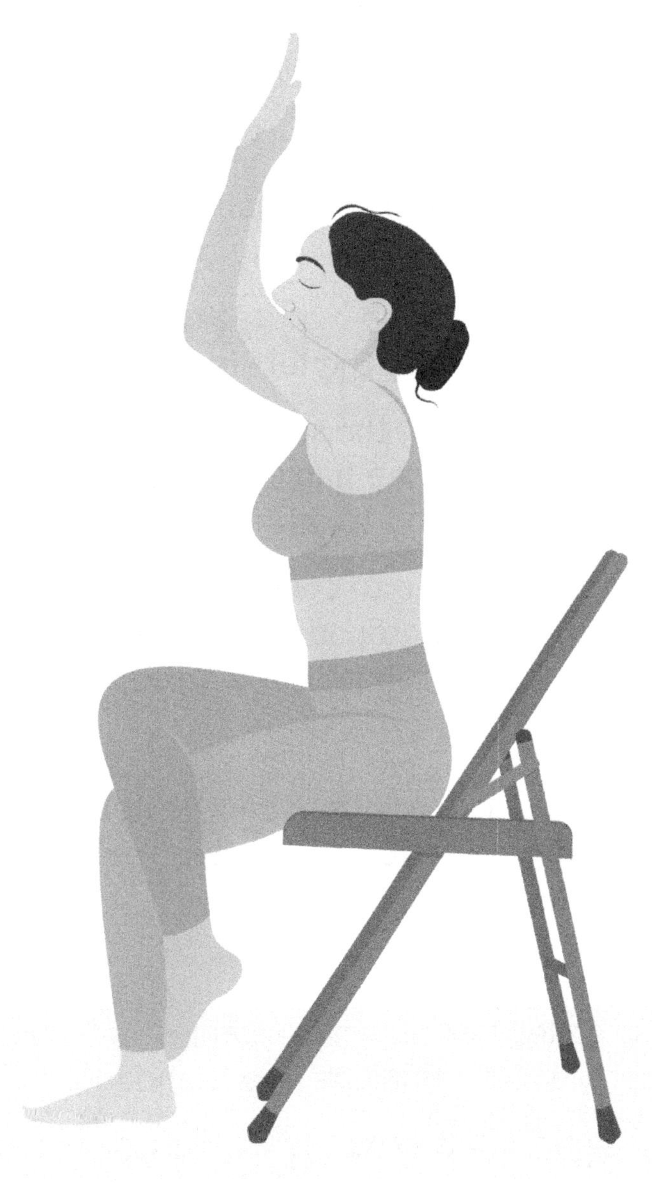

Virabhadrasana II

Even the warrior sometimes rests but, despite being performed in a seated version, this is not the case.

To perform this position first of all the chair must be without armrests, otherwise it is not really possible.

From the basic position we bring the right leg to point with the foot and knee tothe right, about 90 degrees from the left leg which remains stationary.

Once the opening has been found, the seat must be moved slightly to the left insuch a way as to find us with the hamstring and the right buttock resting on theseat instead of with both buttocks.

According to our possibility we go to completely extend the left leg keeping bothfeet well supported on the ground and actively pushing. Do not remain passive in the chair, it is a help but never a support on which to abandon oneself.

Once we have found a good position on the legs, we try to close the abdominalswell, push the coccyx forward "pelvis retroversion" and, as always, stretch the back upwards.

The game is almost done, now all that remains is to raise the arms to the level of the shoulders, which remain relaxed, and look to the right hand.

The position is the same in all respects as Warrior II from standing except that part of your weight is on the chair, it depends on you how much, but try to activate your legs and feel, as you strengthen the muscles, that in reality the chair at some point may not even be there anymore.

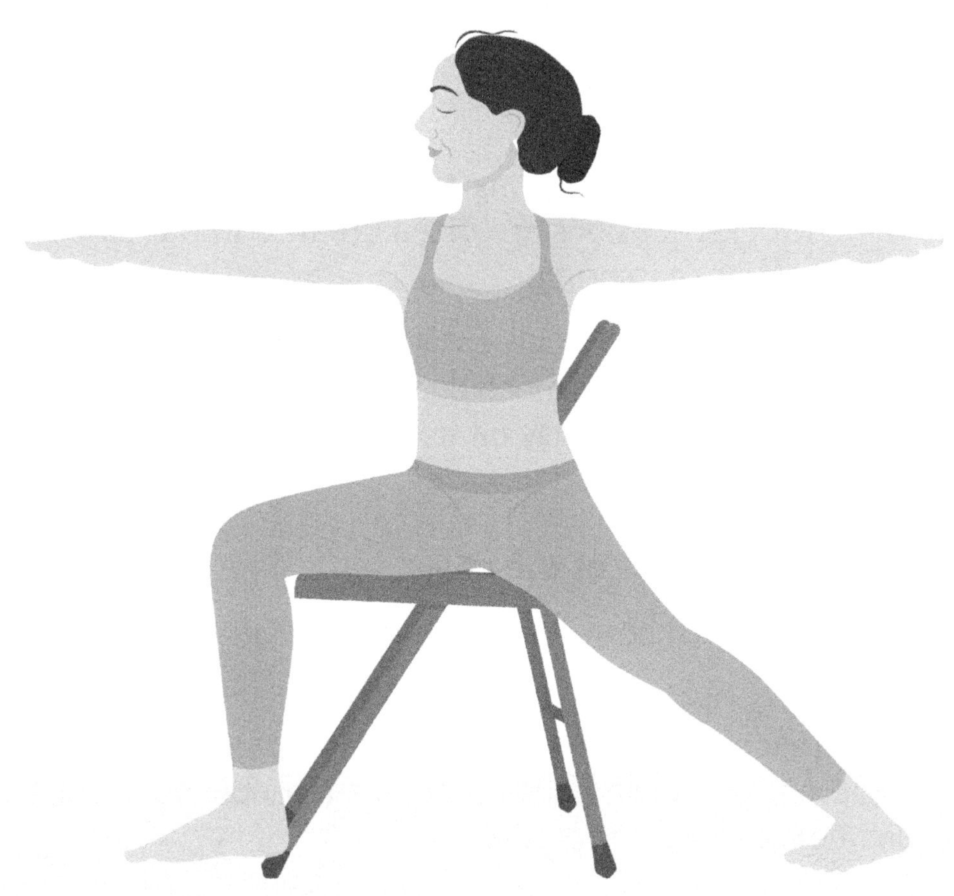

Urdvha mukha Svanasana on the chair

Upward-looking dog is often a difficult position, especially for those suffering from back pain.

If you do not have the ability to bring the pelvis into retroversion without contracting the buttocks, tensions are often created in the lumbar area that arenot at all pleasant or reassuring.

Then you can try this version, much easier to perform with less arching of the spine. Although this version is much lighter than the original one, for many it canstill be challenging, so go easy on it.

Place both hands on the seat of the chair.

Take a long step back with both feet so that your full body weight is resting on your hands.

The arms are extended and the hands and shoulders push down well, the neck must come out of the shoulders and stretch upwards. Don't stay with your neck sunk between your shoulders.

In this version the feet do not rest on the back but remain pointed as they musthold most of the body weight.

Stretch your legs well, look for the retroversion of the pelvis, that is, push the coccyx forward, close the abdominals well and stretch the back upwards.

Look upwards.

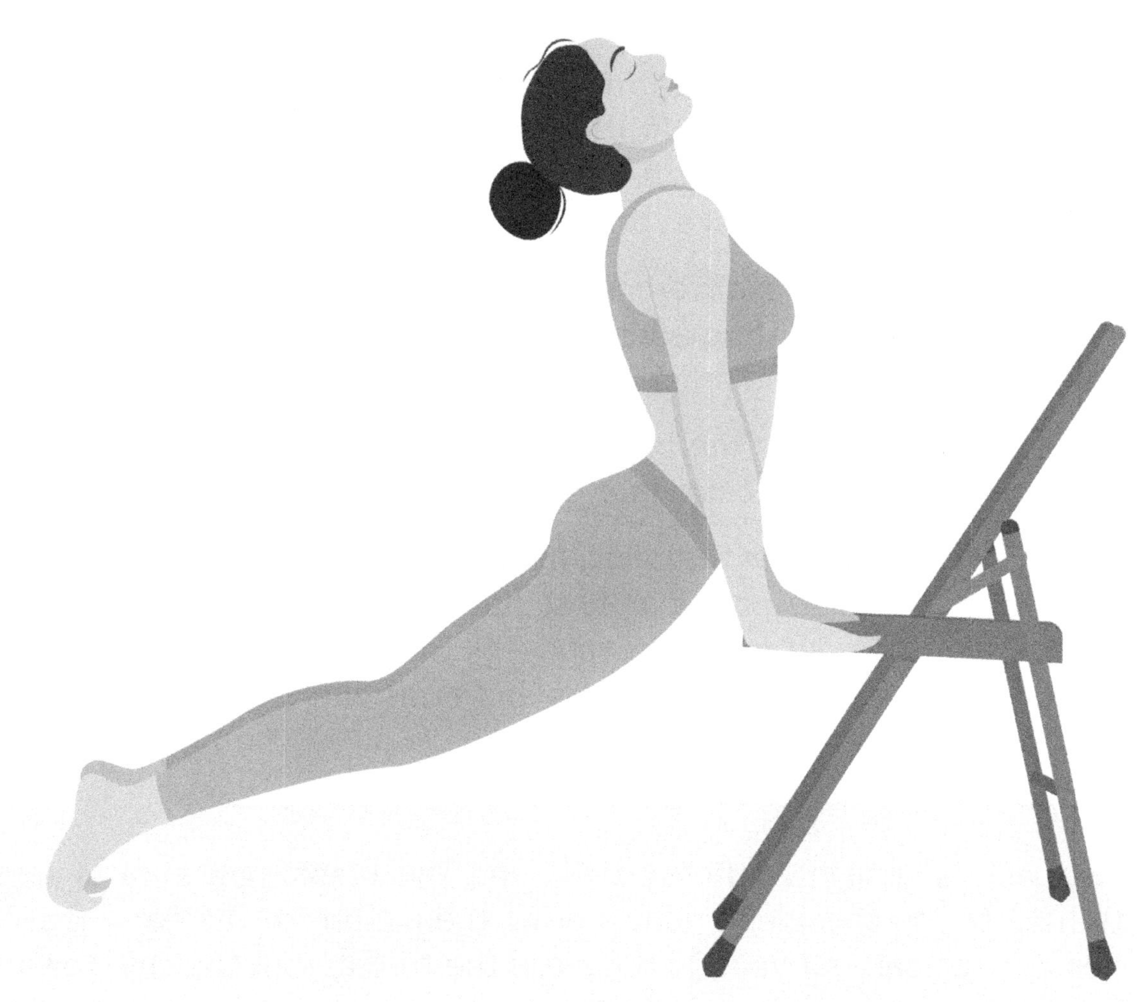

CHAPTER 6 MEDITATION ON THE CHAIR

And here is the time to dedicate ourselves to meditation on the chair.

First of all, know that, meditating sitting on a chair does not detract from the practice compared to meditation with crossed legs or kneeling. In fact, I often encounter the limiting belief that meditation sitting on a chair is a postural adaptation that takes away part of the meaning from the practice.

What really makes the difference is the convenience of the location. A meditation practice performed in an uncomfortable position for your body is counterproductive to the practice itself.

The best meditation is the one you do in an optimal postural condition because it allows you to contact yourself in peace.

To practice meditation in the chair, make sure you keep your back away from the back of the chair and your feet flat on the ground. Leave your arms relaxedand place your hands on your legs to find a position that allows you to release tension in your shoulders and arms with enough muscle tone to maintain a sittingposition.

Your back is straight, but not stiff, and the diaphragm area is free. Pay attentionto the shoulders: do not bring them close to the ears, leave them open as necessary for you. Do not close the throat with the chin towards the chest and do not arch the neck.

The characteristic of this position compared to the previous two (kneeling and crossed legs) is mainly in the support of the feet on the ground. In this case, thesensation of grounding, which comes from the contact of your feet with the floor,can be an additional point to focus attention during the practice.

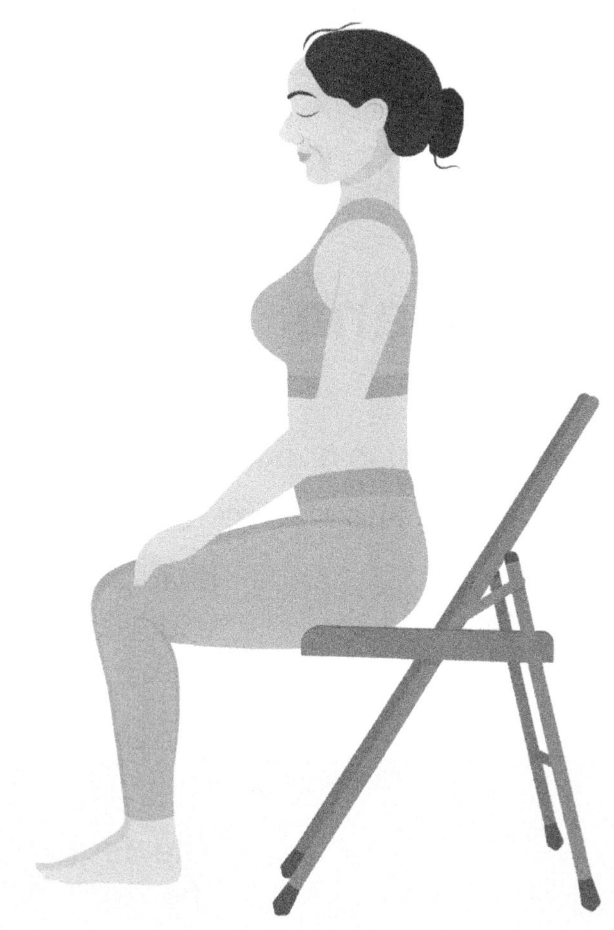

Once you have chosen the best position for your body, it is time to learn to be with what is inside and outside of you, one breath after another.

Using a chair is a great alternative to sitting on the floor if your legs tire easily. However, the risk is that of letting oneself go to an excessive relaxation of the muscles and therefore losing concentration. To avoid this danger, simply sit near the edge of the chair, keeping your back straight. A pillow can be used to help the spine stay erect. The hips should be slightly higher than the knees so as not to slip.

Keep the soles of your feet firmly on the floor.

If you are much taller or shorter than average, you can compensate for this by using a pillow under your feet (for those who are very short) or under the buttocks (for those who are tall).

The hands can be held on the thighs, or folded over the bell

CHAPTER 7 EXERCISES TO LOSE WEIGHT THAT ARE ALSO GOOD FOR THE BACK

Urdhva hastasana

Also known as the raised arms position or palm position. It is useful for stretching the muscles of the arms and abdomen. It is performed as follows:

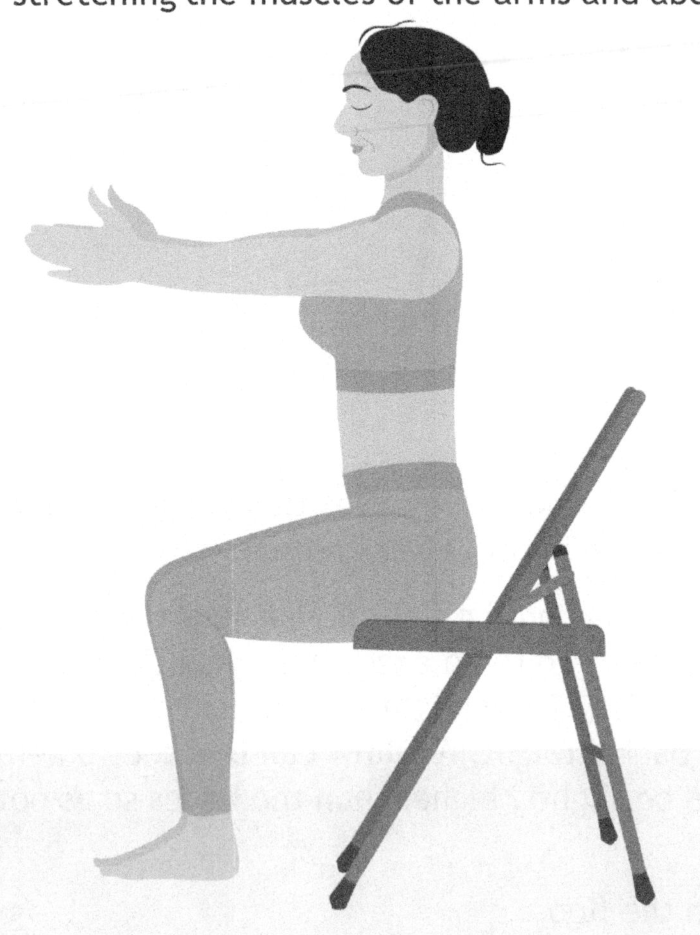

Maintain a natural posture, with your back straight, shoulders relaxed and chest open.

Put your arms on the sides of the chair.

The feet should be parallel to the front and naturally open.

Raise your arms without bending your elbow, so that they are in front of you. Hold them up for a few seconds and then bring them back to the starting position.

If you wish, you can alternate this exercise by raising your hips.

The gaze must be fixed forward to avoid the accumulation of tension on the cervix. Breathe deeply and slowly, without hastening the movement so as not to compromise the posture of the back. Yoga positions have varying degrees of complexity, so they must be adjusted according to the physical condition of each.

Ardha matsyendrasana

Also known as the half twist position, it is suitable for those suffering from back pain. Its original version is performed sitting on the floor, but is adapted to yoga with the chair for the elderly as follows:

Sit sideways in the chair, with your whole body facingright.

Stretch your back, bring your feettogether and create some tension in the abdomen.

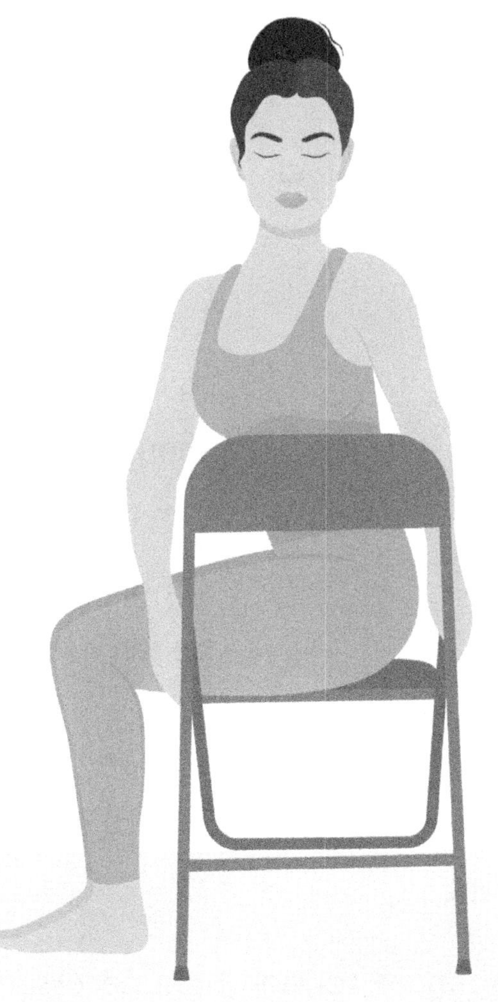

Slowly rotate your uppertorso until you face the backof the chair.

If possible, try not to liftyour legs off the ground andkeep your hips still.

Hold your back with your hands to complete themovement. Hold the tensionfor a few seconds and then return to the starting position.

After 5-10 repetitions, switch sides and repeat withthe other side of the body.

Utthita parsvakonasana

Known in the traditional variation as an extended lateral angle, this position is perfect for stretching all the back muscles. It requires a greater degree of flexibility and is accomplished as follows:

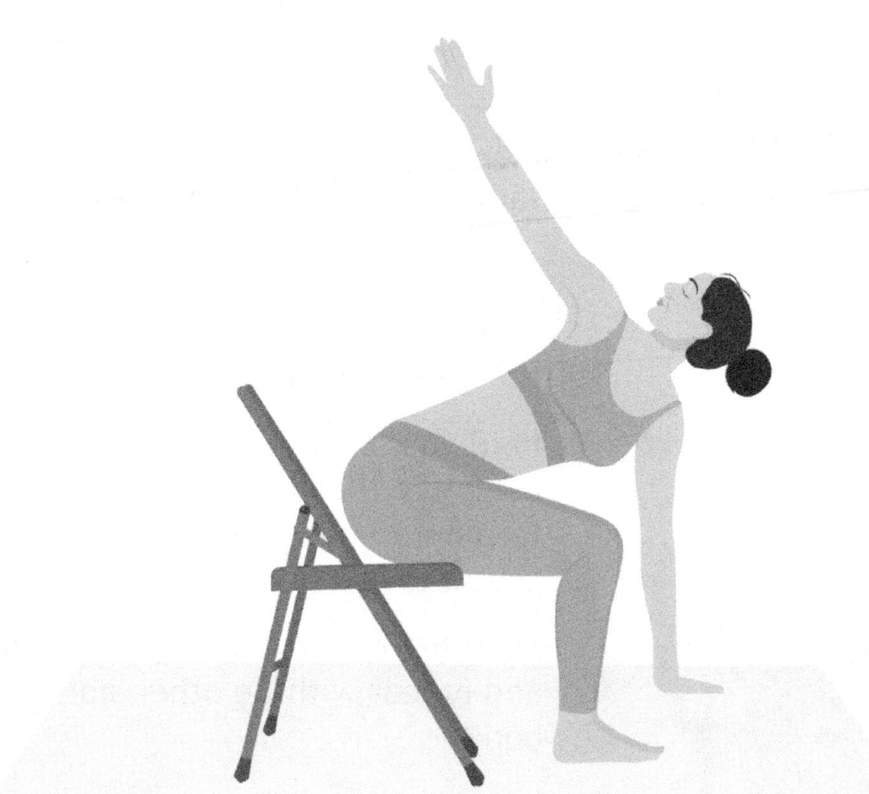

Sit in a natural position with your arms extended to the sides.Lean your body to the left, bring it forward and touch the floor with the palm of your right hand. The arm should be fully extended and the contact base should be an inch or two above the left foot.

Fully extend the other arm, the left one, upward and fix your gaze on it. **Watch your back while doing the movement.**

Make sure it is straight and that there is no more tension than necessary.After holding the position for several seconds, switch sides.

Uttanasana

Finally, the position of the clamp or uttanasana cannot be missing.

Sit in the starting position with your arms extended at your sides.

Slowly lower yourself forward paying attention to your backand directing your gaze straight ahead.

Touch the floor with your palms and hold this position for a few seconds.

Shoulders should be facing forward, arms fully extended, and heels should not lift off the ground.

If you can't, you can only use your fingers as a contact surface, although you should keep in mind that this increases the stress on your back.

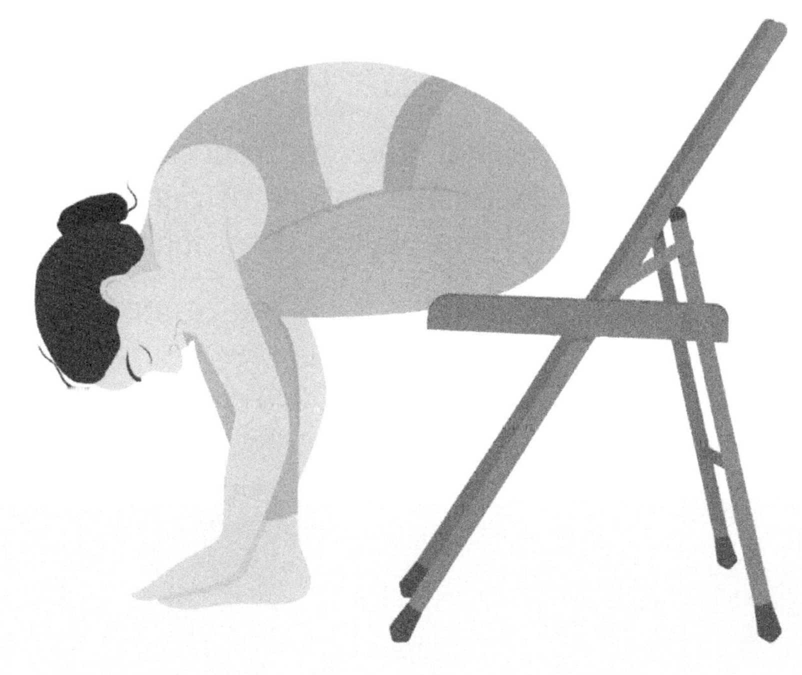

Switch sides

Sit sideways on the chair with your legs to the right.

If your feet aren't touching the ground, use blocks to support

them.Begin to rotate with your torso to the right,

and squeeze the back of the chair with your hands.

Keep your hips aligned with your knees and feet as you push with your right handand pull with your left.

You will feel a sense of openness around the middle of the back.

Stretch the spine from the coccyx to the top of the skull. Now bring your attention to the breath.

As you breathe in, imagine yourself expanding and getting bigger, as if you wereexpanding the limits of your breath.

As you exhale, rotate and release any stress or any other resistance you are feeling. Hold for 3 long, full breaths.

When we feel tired, compressed and contracted, it is really helpful to breathe in and regain the expansive nature of our freest and most joyful state: the vibration of youth. Keep paying attention to your breath.

Then, loosen the posture and repeat it on the other

side.Do this pose 2 times on each side.

When you repeat it for the second time, observe how you are most likely able torotate deeper because you have softened your back and loosened some of the resistance.

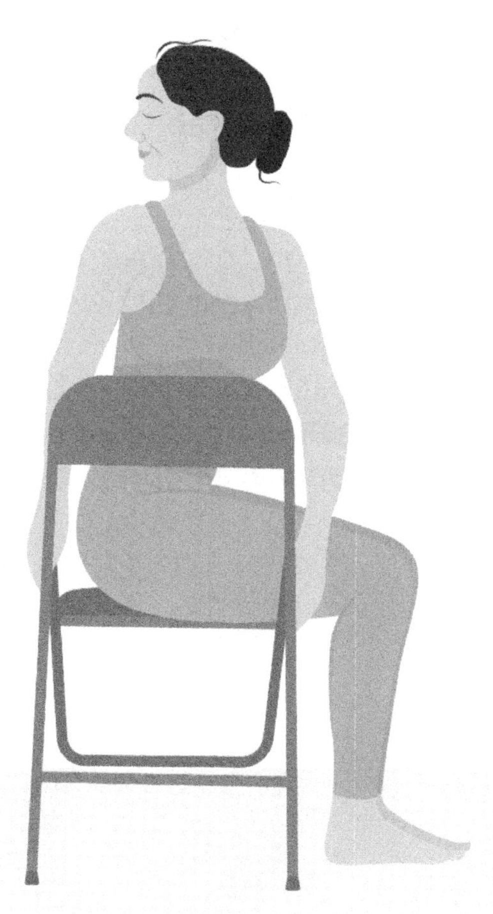

Shoulder stretch with chair

Sit on the chair and squeeze the edge of the seat with your fingers pointing in the same direction as your knees.

Slide off the seat and bring your buttocks down,keeping them off the ground.

Let the central part of the spine (at the level of the lower ends of the shoulderblades) press on the edge of the seat.

Extend your arms behind you, and grab the top of the backrest.In this position,

the upper arms rotate outward.

Keep your hands in this position, or move them downwards by tightening thelower grips of the chair, until your elbows are pointing upwards.

Let the hips drop, and the seat press against the lower ends of the shoulder blades. If the edge of the chair is sharp, place a blanket over the seat.
Now breathe, letting the heart area open, also favoring the opening of the central part of the spine.

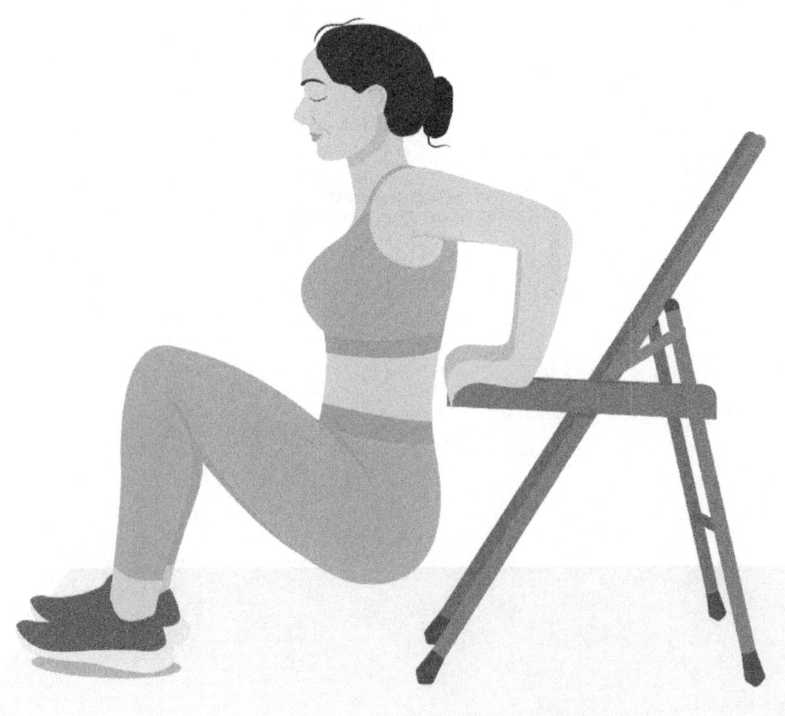

Salamba Sarvangasana (Candle Pose with support, with chair)

Place a blanket on the seat and stack a few at the foot of the chair.
Sit facing the backrest.
Bring your legs over it and lean back, placing your hands on the blankets on the ground.

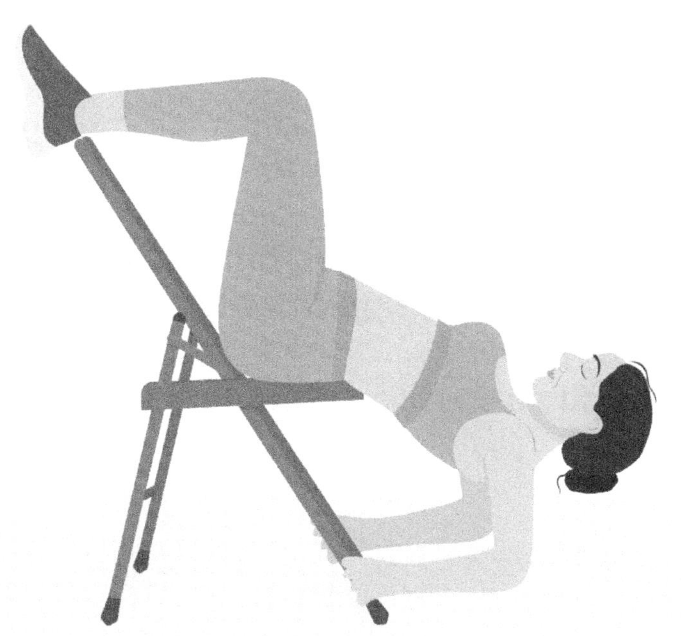

To lie down, grab the sides of the seat first and then the legs of the chair as you rest your sacrum on the seat and your shoulders on the blankets on the floor.
If necessary, place a blanket under your head.
Extend your arms and grab the back legs of the chair. Begin lifting the heart area. Extend your legs against the backrest.Now give yourself a moment of rest. Let your breath go completely, close your eyes and relax.Stay in position for at least 5 minutes.

With practice, you can go up to 20 minutes.
To get out of the position, let go of your hands and bend your knees.
Place your feet on the seat, and use your arms to crawl back onto the blankets.
Rest your buttocks on the blankets, and let your calves rest on the seat.
Lie on your back with your arms above your head.

CHAPTER 8 RECOVER ENERGY AND CONCENTRATION

Is it possible to practice yoga without unrolling a mat?

A chair is enough to be able to perform some suitable positions to recharge yourenergy and to improve the levels of mindfulness. Using a chair as a support can be a good alternative to being able to practice yoga despite some impediments.The difficulties can be linked to a physical limit, or to the lack of space for a classic and traditional practice, or because there is little time available.

Yoga on a chair is indicated for example in the office, when a decrease in attention is perceived. 10-15 minutes are enough to relax the mind and reactivate the body. It is also suitable for students, since the execution of certainpositions allows you to reactivate the energies, bringing the mind back to a stateof greater concentration. Chair yoga is specifically suitable for those with a disability, or with back or leg ailments.

The classic postures of yoga are modified and adapted to be performed thanks to the help of this support.

BENEFITS

Yoga on the chair allows you to:

- Relax the mind;
- Reactivate the psychophysical energies;
- Stimulate the muscles of the legs and arms;
- Relieve tension in the shoulders and back;
- Improve joint mobility;
- Favor greater balance;
- Re-oxygenate body and mind thanks to conscious breathing.

What asanas to perform

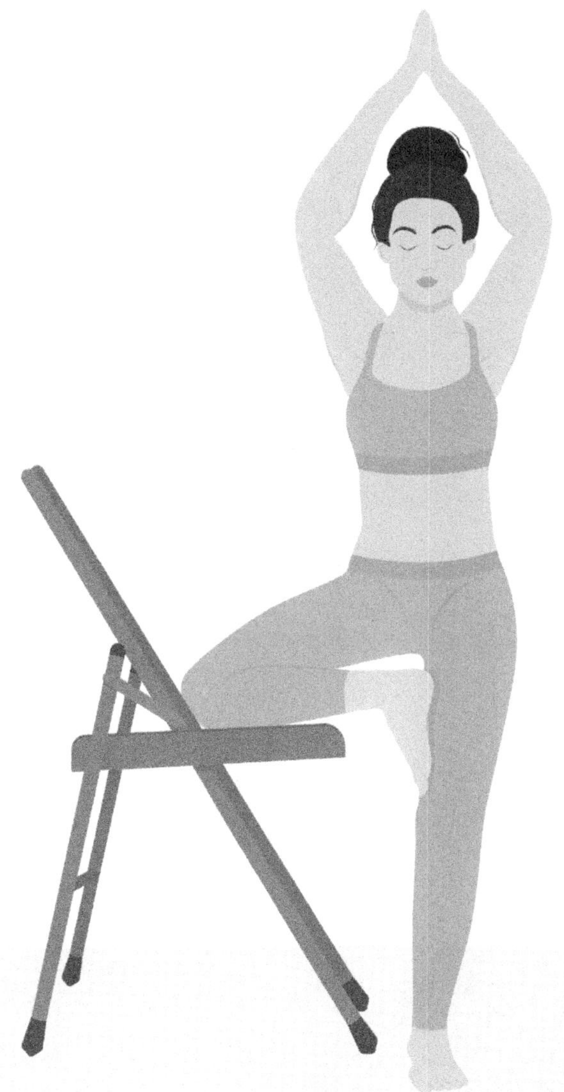

There are numerous yoga positions that can be changed slightly, so that you can practice them on the chair.

Vrikshasana (the position of the tree): it is indicated for examplefor beginners who, for the first performances, can use the chair as a support.

Utthita Trikonasana (the position of the triangle), Utthita Parsvakonasana (extended lateral angle position) andArdha Matsyendrasana (half position of Matsyendra): thanks to the use of the chair these postures can also be performed by those with motor difficulties.

Among the first masters to introduce supports - including the use of the chair - into yoga practice was BKS Iyengar. He stated that:

"Disease is created when the energy does not move".

Therefore, also through this adaptation of the practice we have the opportunityto better circulate the energies, thus reactivating the mind and body.

WARNING: As with any yoga style, also in this case it is necessary to start practicing with an expert teacher, capable of explaining in detail how to performthe postures using the chair as a support.

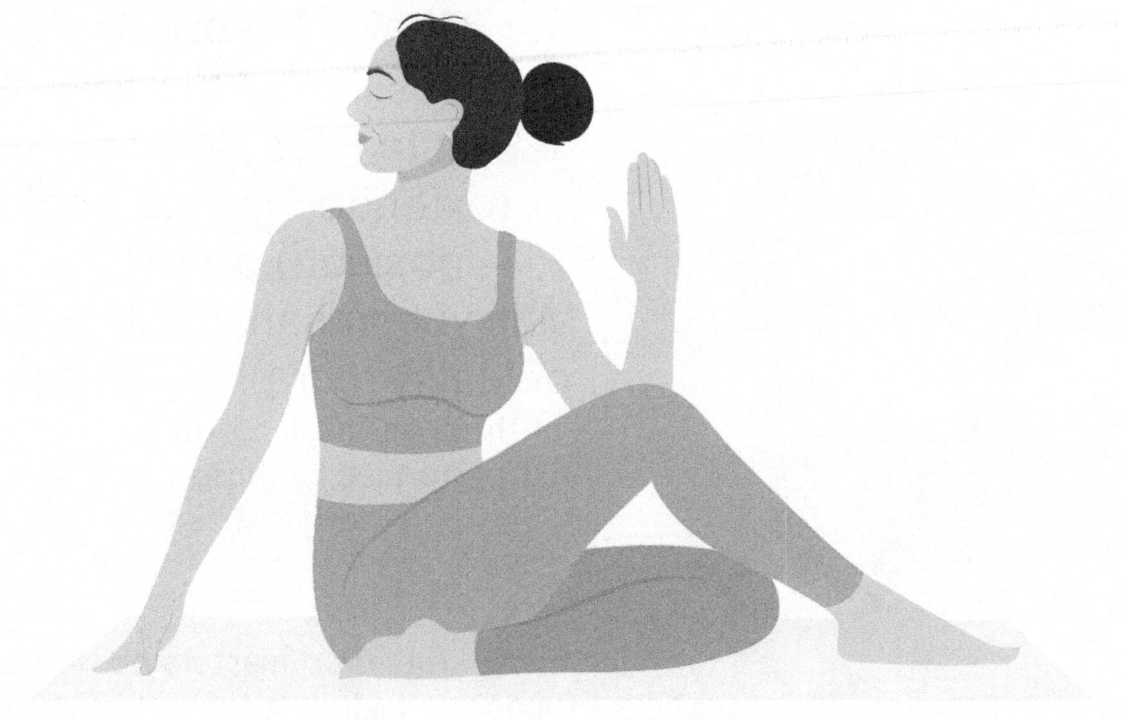

CHAPTER 9 PARIVRTTA PARSVAKONASANA THE ANTI-CELLULITE ASANA ON A CHAIR

While sitting, and therefore with suitable support even for the most sedentary, you can perform the lateral angle in torsion, which squeezes out stagnant liquidsand toxins.

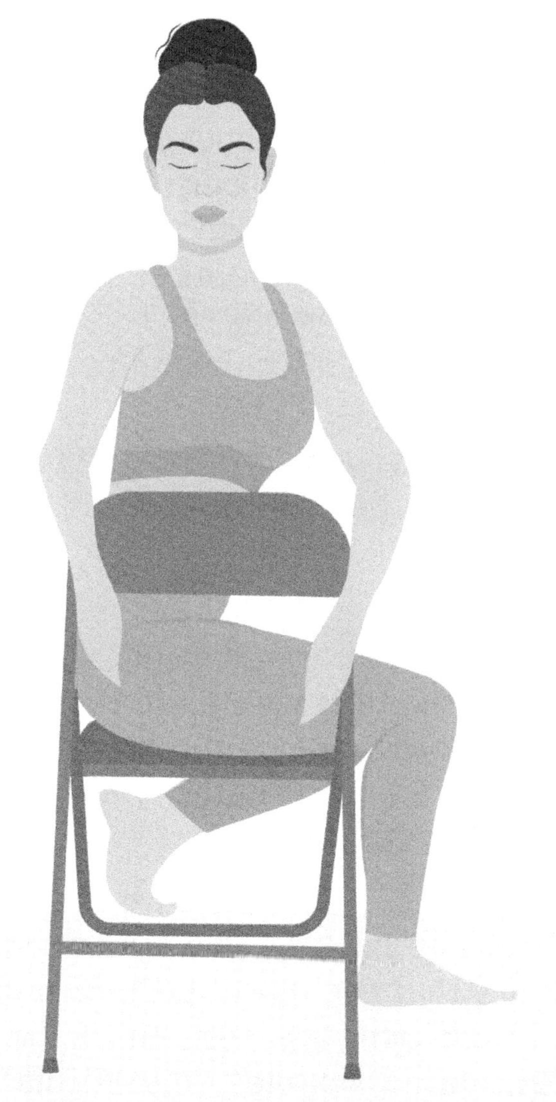

Many women have never tried yoga, for fear of not being sufficiently capable and not being able to reach and hold the poses correctly.

A very suitable asana for performing on the chair is the Side Angle Twisting (Parivrtta Parsvakonasana). The chair must have a flat seat and a height that allows you to keep your feet flat on the ground and your knees bent at 90 degrees.

HOW IT IS DONE

Sit so that the backrest is on your right side. Extend your left leg back, so that it comes off the supporting surface, and twist your torso to the right. Suck the navel towards the spine, to protect the lower back, and grab the back of the chair, to help you hold the pose. Stay for 5-6 full breaths and repeat the exerciseon the other side.

CHAPTER 10 YOGA: THE PIGEON POSE ON A CHAIR TO RELEASE TENSIONS

A sedentary lifestyle causes muscle contractures, blocks, stiffness and postural disharmony. Yoga is a great antidote andthere are effective asanas that you can perform while sitting

When you sit for a long time and do not engage in any motor activity, it is easy to feel localized muscular tension and annoying pains, because you assume forced, unbalanced and often unnatural positions. This creates contractures in the neck, shoulders and back, which negatively affect the postural structure, concentration and mood, but the yoga teacher Francesca Cassia explains that there are very effective asanas to re-harmonize the posture and mobilize the joints. Indeed, some can also be performed while sitting on a chair, so they arewithin the reach of anyone, even the most sedentary and those who are out of practice. One of these is the Pigeon pose (Raja Kapotasana), which on the chairis slightly modified compared to the version on the mat.

You can also resort to yoga several times a day: you don't need to spend a lot oftime on the pose, small breaks are enough, but the rebalancing effects on posture and muscle tension are immediate.

How it is done

Sit on the chair and bring the ankle of one leg over the thigh of the other. You have to place it just above the knee, with the tibia parallel to the ground, so that it makes a figure. Flex the torso forward, keeping the hands clasped in frontof the chest, and hold the position for 5-6 full breaths. Then repeat the asana onthe other side, reversing the position of the legs.

Stop bowing

The exercise mobilizes the hips and reduces back fatigue by extending the spine.It therefore contrasts the tendency that one has to become bent over, when oneis sitting for a long time. In addition, the position of the legs is particularly effective for stretching the gluteus muscles, in particular it acts on the piriformis, which is a muscle located in the center of the buttock, very small butvery insidious: in fact, it has a tendency to contract easily and presses on the sciatic nerve, with sometimes painful outcomes.

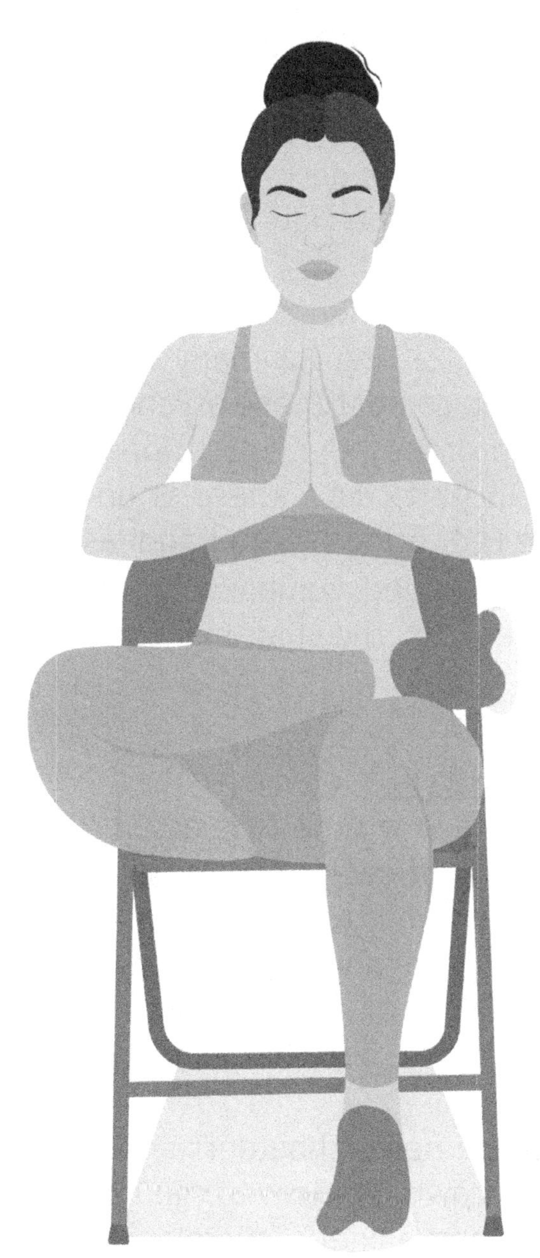

CHAPTER 11 YOGA: THE HALF BRIDGE ASANA

Stationary on the sofa or sitting at a desk, you find yourself contracted, tense and in a bad mood: the pose of the Half Bridge, performed on a chair, is a medicine for the body and the mind.
It happens to everyone, on days when one is more sedentary and forced to stay at home for a long time, sitting for many hours: one feels tense, sore, nervous and not very lucid. To combat these psychophysical ailments, the yoga teacher Francesca Cassia proposes the execution of asanas chosen ad hoc, with the helpof a chair. In particular, there is one that proves to be very effective: the layingof the Half bridge (Setu Bandhasana).
The execution is slightly modified compared to that on the mat and the presenceof the support offered by the chair makes the asana within everyone's reach.

<u>The risks of a sedentary lifestyle</u>
Staying on a sofa or chair for a long time, one assumes an unbalanced posture, in which the harmonious play of reciprocal tensions between the muscles is altered. One is led to sag, to bend, to close the shoulders: the spine loses its natural curves and the diaphragm also stiffens, with the result that breathing isshortened. The flexor muscles of the legs (ileo-psoas) shorten, leading to stiffness in the hips and back pain, because their upper insertion is at the level of the lumbar vertebrae.
Result? Localized pains in the neck, shoulders and back, less lucidity (due to thegeneral circulatory slowdown and less oxygenation of all tissues) and the appearance of nervousness and anxiety, correlated with shorter and blocked breathing. The Half Bridge asana counteracts all these annoyances.

HOW TO PERFORM THE HALF BRIDGE ASANA

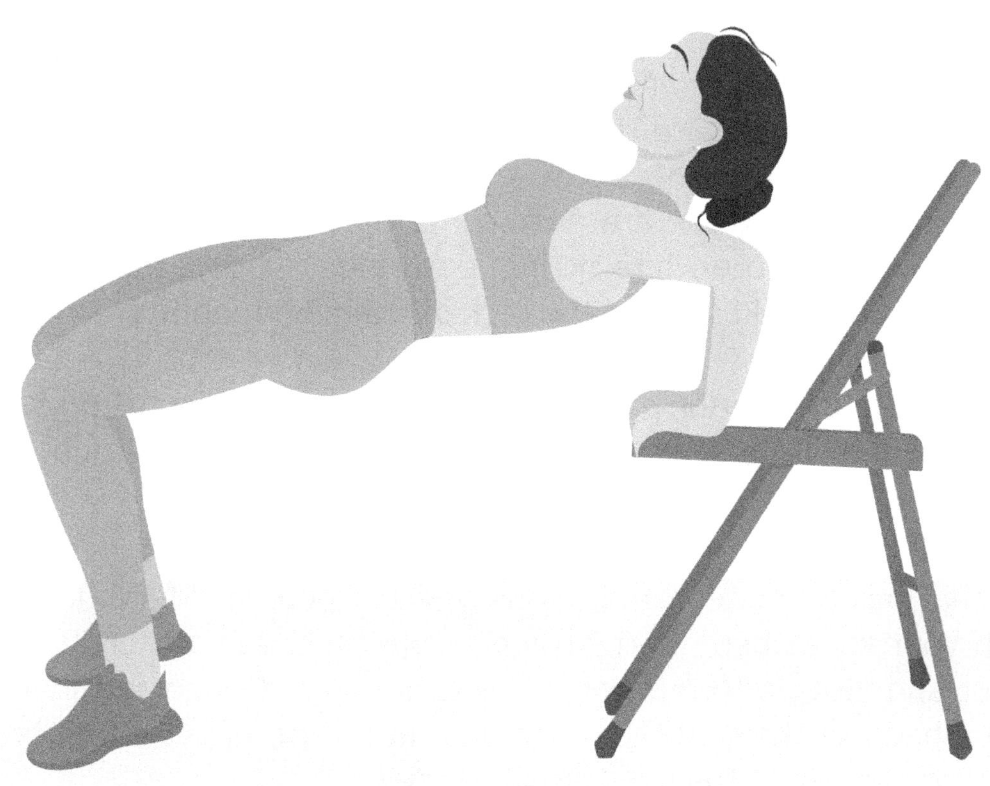

In the execution on the ground, it is very similar to the Pilates bridging, but the arching of the back that characterizes it can also be reproduced on a chair. Placeyour hands on the outer edges of the seat and extend your legs, keeping the solesof your feet on the ground. Then lift your hips and arch your whole body back. Ifyou find it difficult, there is a simplified variant, in which you just have to archyour back a little, without lifting your buttocks from the chair.

his arching of the spine mobilizes it, dissolving its stiffness. The extension of the anterior muscle chain is very useful for relaxing the ileo-psoas whose lengthening, according to the yogi masters, is a source of calm and lucidity. Finally, by opening the chest, lung capacity increases and breathing becomes deeper, all to the advantage of tissue oxygenation and a pleasant anti-stress effect.

CHAPTER 12 MATSYENDRASANA IN A CHAIR

Twisting asanas stimulate the lymphatic system and some, thanks to the supportoffered by a chair, are really within anyone's reach

Talking about yoga positions of torsion can bring to mind images of practitioners with an extraordinarily articulated physique, who perform contortionist movements and are therefore unsuitable for the general public. It is actually a misleading thought, because there are asanas of this type within everyone's reach. Indeed, there are even some that can be carried out with the help of a chair, therefore while sitting, ensuring a support that facilitates the execution and that makes up for the lack of training, mobility, and muscle strength.

Blood and lymphatic circulation slow down, causing stagnation of liquids and toxins, when the lifestyle is sedentary: but yoga can be a valid antidote.

HOW IT IS DONE

Get a chair that has a flat seat and allows you to keep your feet flat on the ground, with your knees bent at right angles. Sit on the chair, cross one leg overthe other and also perform a torso twist, helping (if necessary) with the supportof one hand to the seat itself. Remain in position for 5-6 full breaths and then repeat the whole thing on the other side.

SURPRISING BENEFITS

The benefits given by such an easy and apparently almost banal pose are surprising and depend on many factors. The anti-retention and detoxifying effectis due to the fact that the lymphatic system is stimulated in depth and the Lord of fish is therefore a pose to be performed as first aid, when imperfections are present, but also to prevent them. That's not all. Since it stretches the entire muscles of the torso, up to the shoulders, Matsyendrasana gives a sense of greatlightness and a more open and elegant posture. Like all poses in which the chestand shoulders open, it expands lung capacity and unlocks the diaphragm, freeingup breathing and making it more complete and deeper. The result is greater oxygenation of the blood and, therefore, of all tissues: this is also an importantelement for improving metabolism and cell renewal, both in critical areas and inany other part of the body.

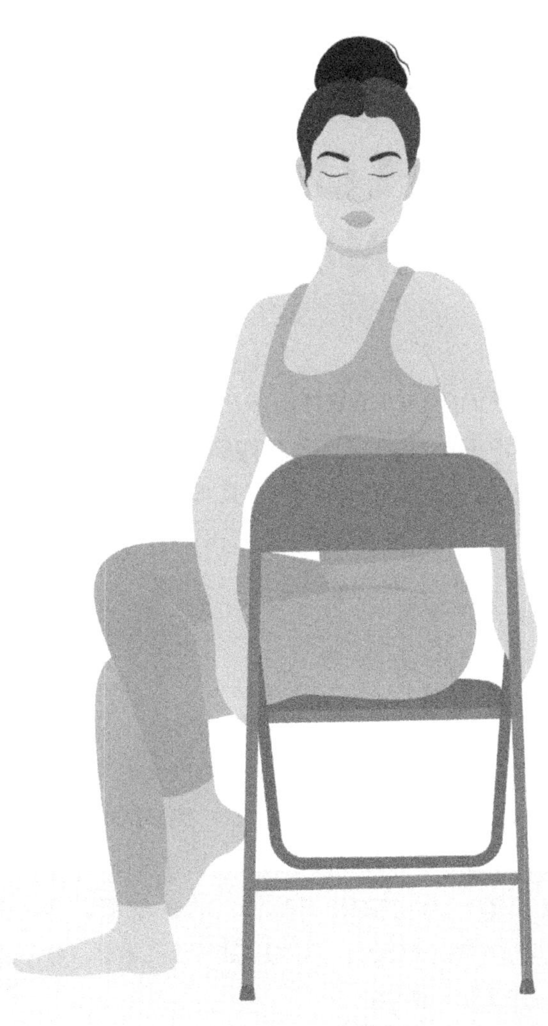

CHAPTER 13 EXERCISES YOU CAN DO WHILE SITTING TO SPEED UP YOUR METABOLISM AND LOSE WEIGHT

Doing physical activity and staying healthy is an imperative that now comes fromseveral fronts in terms of health and psycho-physical well-being. Those who havelittle time to train and plan a workout session could also perform an effective "office gymnastics". Here are 3 exercises you can do while sitting to speed up your metabolism and lose weight.

Those who think that training necessarily requires a gym full of equipment, doesnot know that there are several alternative solutions to keep fit. Even sitting comfortably on a chair, it is possible to perform some workouts that help the body stay healthy and reduce sedentary lifestyle. The 3 exercises that we will illustrate next aim to train each one specific area of the body. Starting from theupper area, shoulders and arms, we follow a short circuit that ends with the training of the legs.

The first exercise

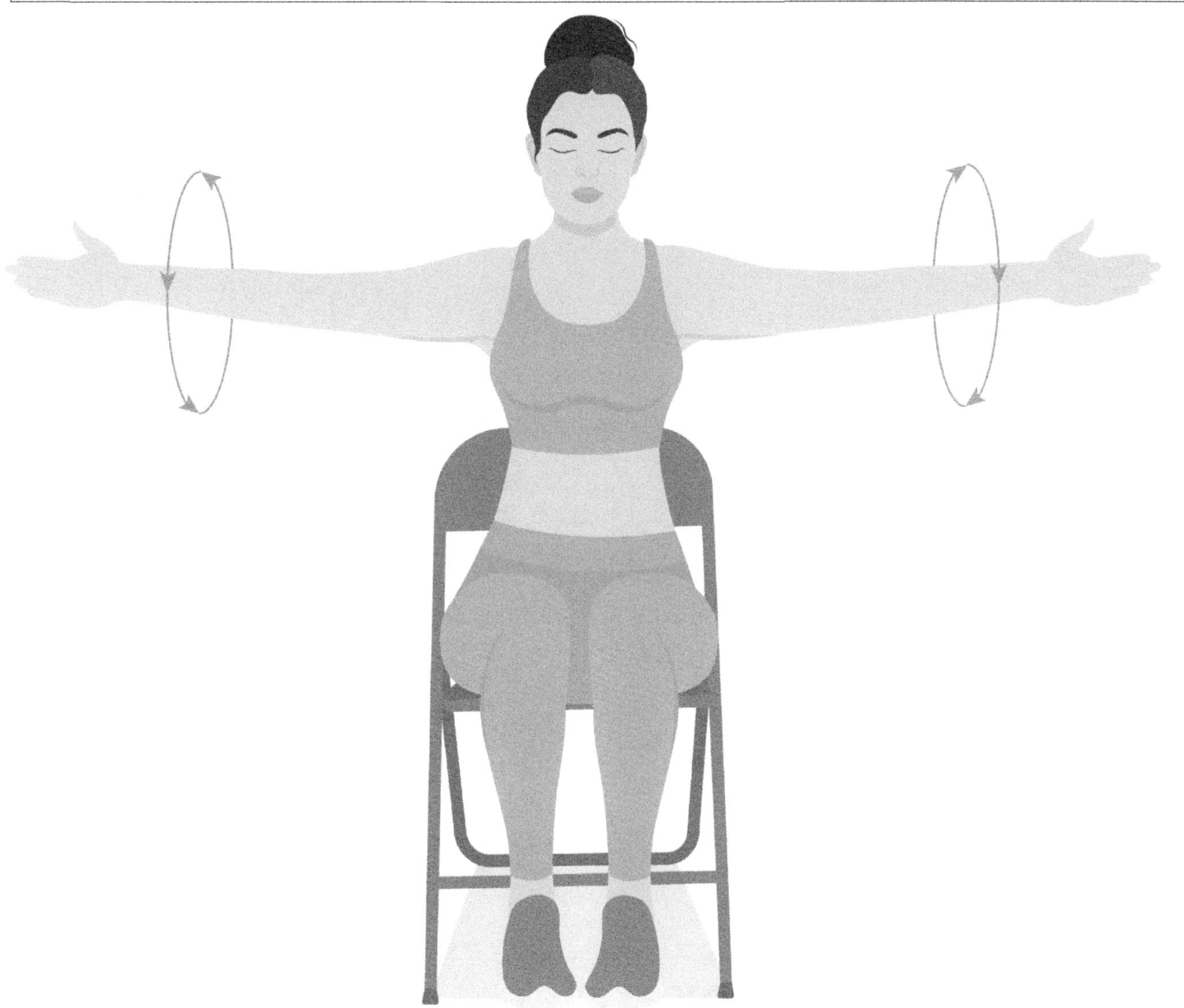

The first exercise that can be done while sitting is the Arm Circles. While seated,extend your arms and keep them straight at shoulder height. Make circular movements in a clockwise and then anticlockwise direction as if to form small circles with the arms. Perform the movement with some rapidity and taking careto keep the muscles of the arms tense. Repeat the series of 20 circles per direction three times. This exercise serves to strengthen the muscles of the armsand shoulders. For even more effective results, keep your core contracted as youperform to strengthen your abdominals.

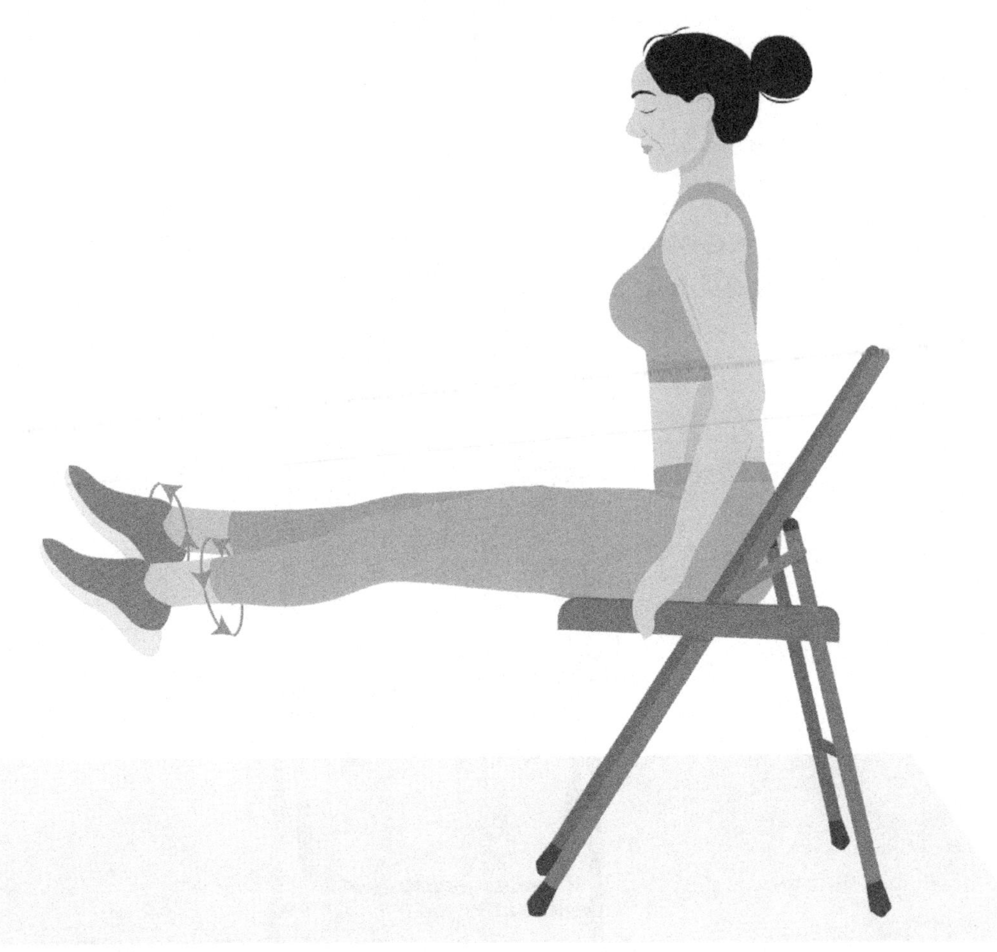

The second exercise

The second exercise that can be performed while seated is the Straight Leg Circles. In this case it is a question of drawing circles, as for the arms, but with the legs. Lifting both legs and placing your hands on the chair, draw small circlesfirst in one direction and then in the opposite. Thanks to this exercise, your legsand abs will be strengthened.

Gluteal Squeeze

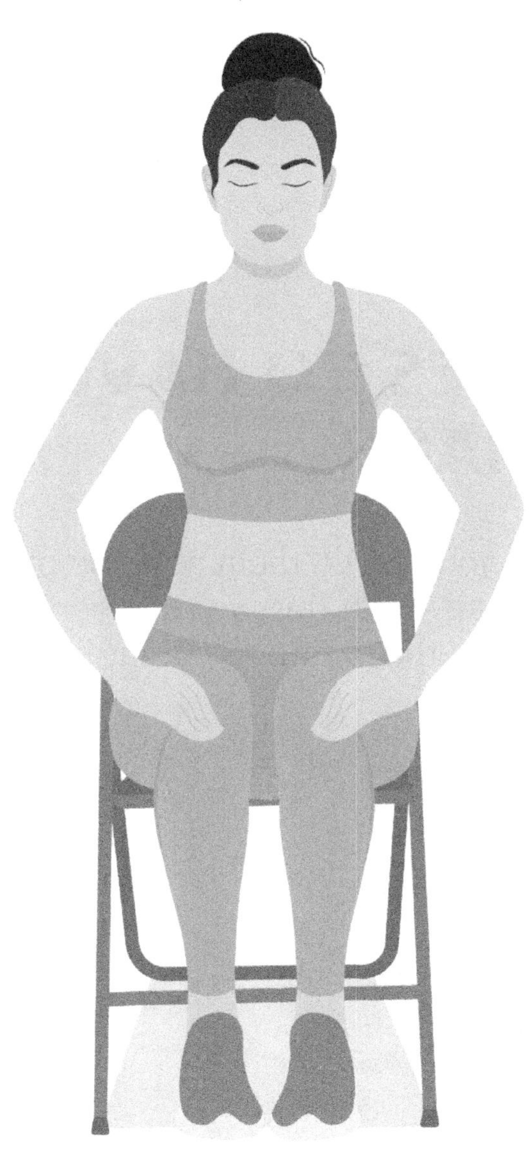

Finally, perform the Gluteal Squeeze. While seated, you simply contract and relax your glutes and hamstrings for at least three sets of 15 repetitions. Strengthening the glutes and hamstring serves to prevent numerous back problems such as lower back pain.

By combining adequate training with a healthy lifestyle and diet, the results of your commitment will certainly not be long in coming.

CHAPTER 14 EXERCISES TO HAVE A FLAT STOMACH

The good thing about these exercises is that you can do them at home or in the office while you work. All you need is a chair. With this, you can perform different sets of exercises in just a few minutes that will be of great help in getting a flat stomach.

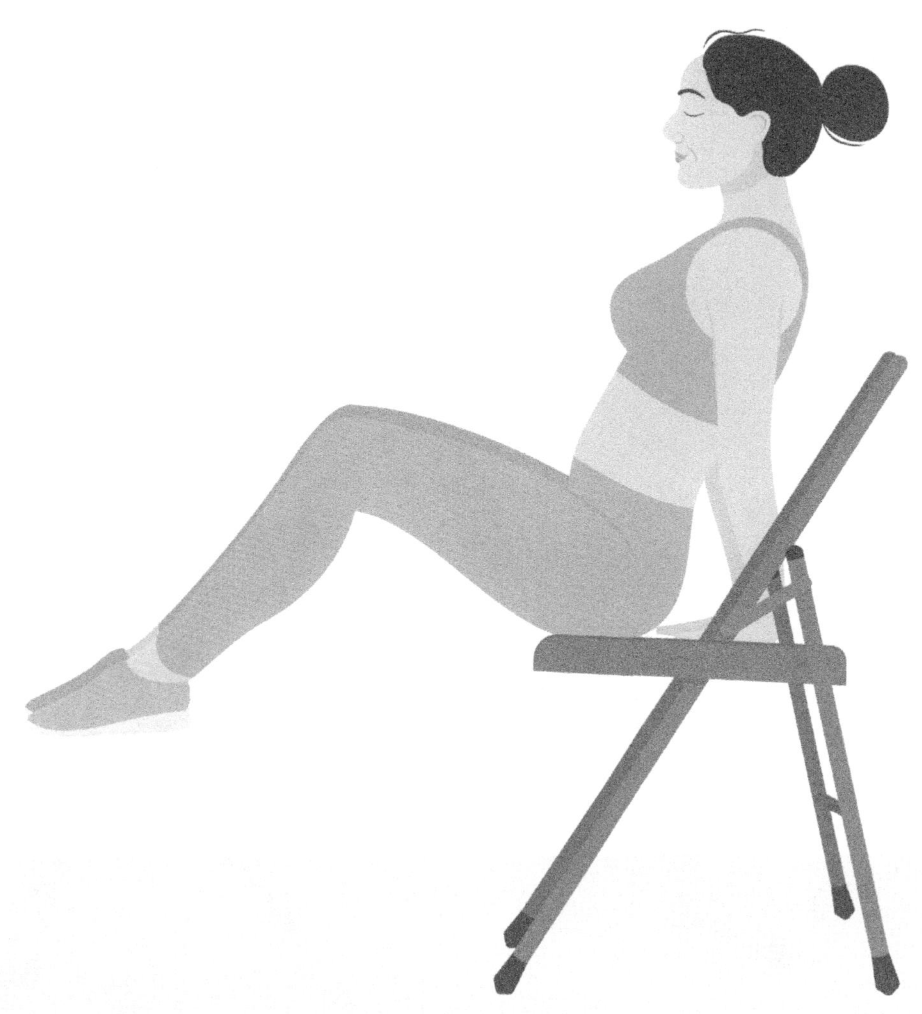

Lift your knees with your body

With this exercise you will be able to shape your waistline and put your abdominal muscles to work. It will help you eliminate the "rolls" that usually appear around the waist.

To do this exercise, you should sit on the edge of the chair and keep your back straight. Then you will grab the armrests and tilt your body to one side, leaning on one of your buttocks. Now you will join your knees and raise them as close toyour chest as possible. Now go back to the starting position and repeat the process about 10 or 20 times for each side.

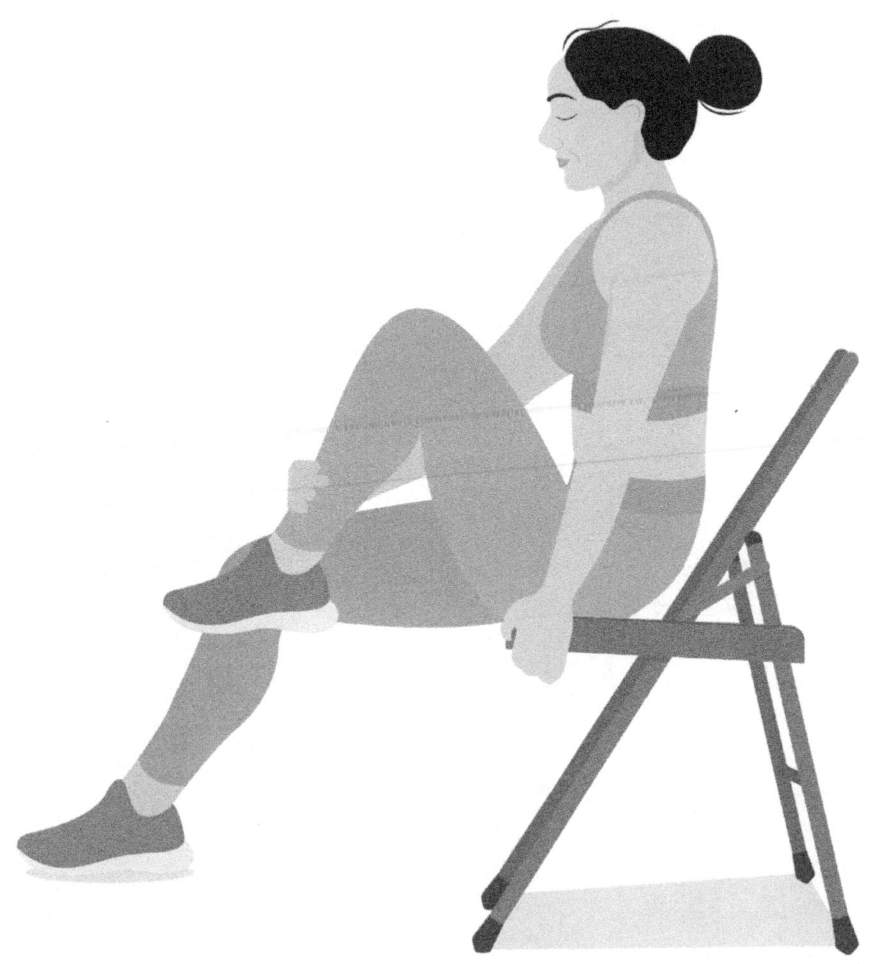

Touch the floor

With this set of exercises, you will get the flat stomach you want and the hip andwaistline in better shape. To do this exercise, you need to turn your body to theright as you lean forward a little. You will be holding your left foot with your right hand. You will hold this position for a few seconds and then return to the starting position. You will repeat the process 20 to 30 times on each side.

Elevation of the knees

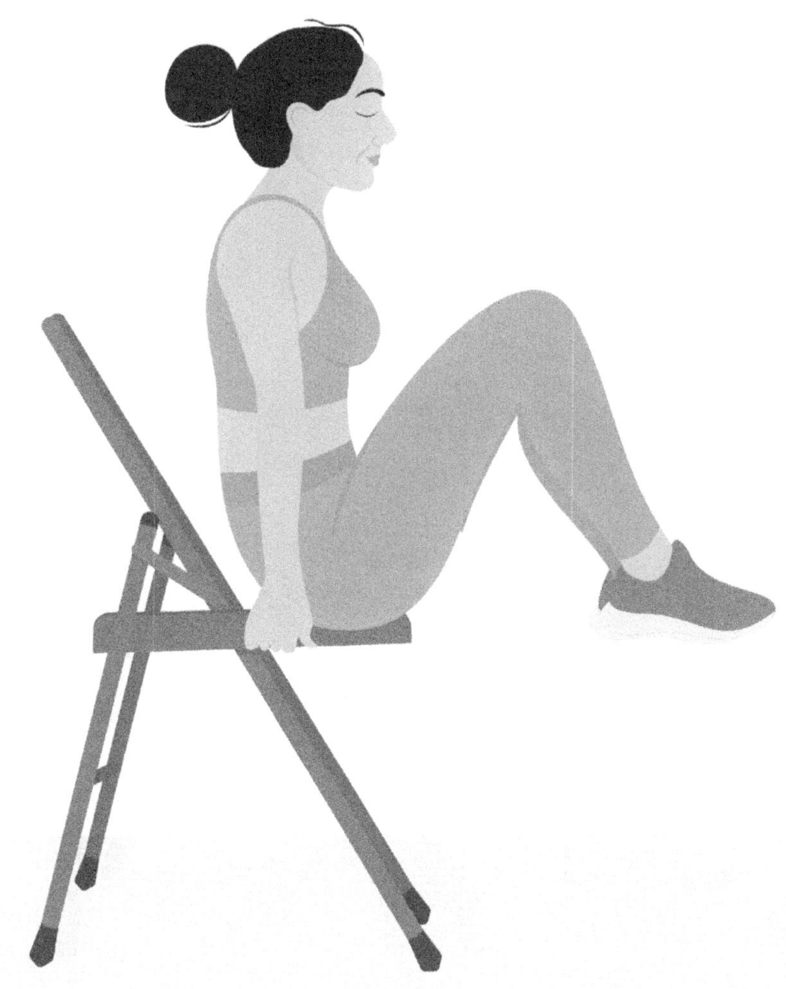

With this exercise you will strengthen the muscles of the abdomen, back and shoulders. To do this, you will need to have a chair with armrests and it shouldn'thave wheels.

To start, sit in the chair and put your arms on the armrests. Now you will lift thebody separating the hip from the chair at the foot of the floor. At the same time,you will use the abdomen to bring the knees to the chest. You will hold this position for about 15 or 20 seconds, and then return to the starting position. Repeat this exercise 4 times on both sides.

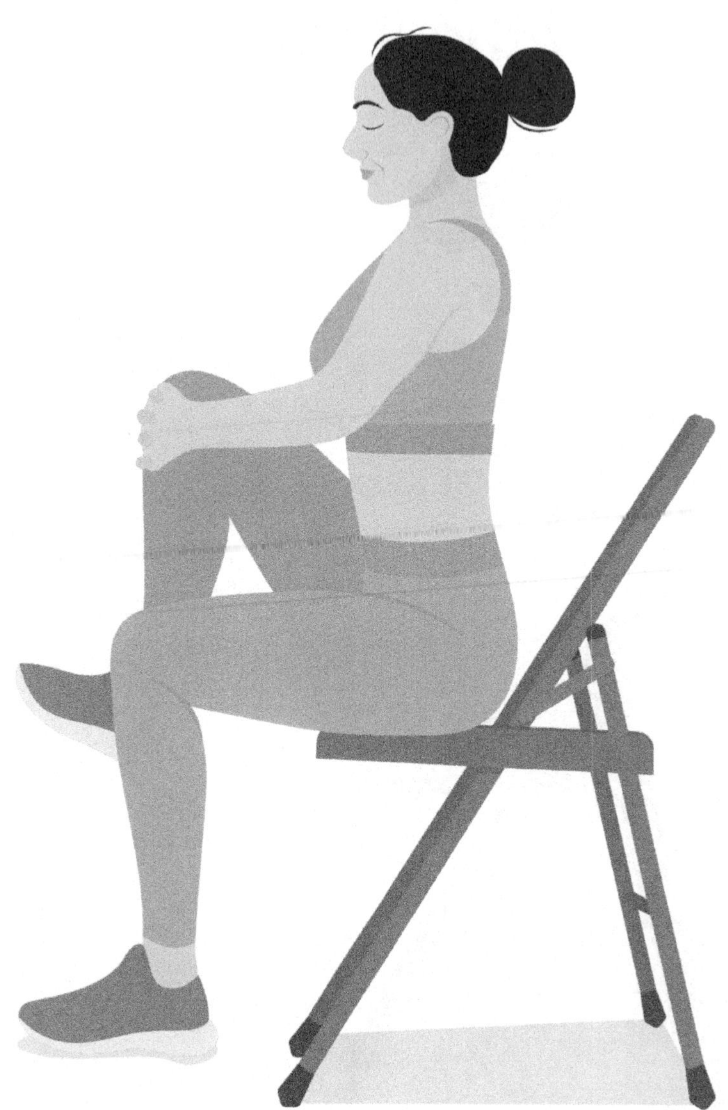

Raise your knees to your chest

Thanks to this exercise,you will get a flat stomach, strengthenyour abdomen and improve digestion. To do this, sit in a chair andkeep your back straight.Now, place your feet in front of you at hip level.With your back straight,lift one knee to your chest. To better stretchthe abdomen, you can hold the knee with yourhands. Then return tothe starting position.Repeat this process 20 to 30 times with both knees.

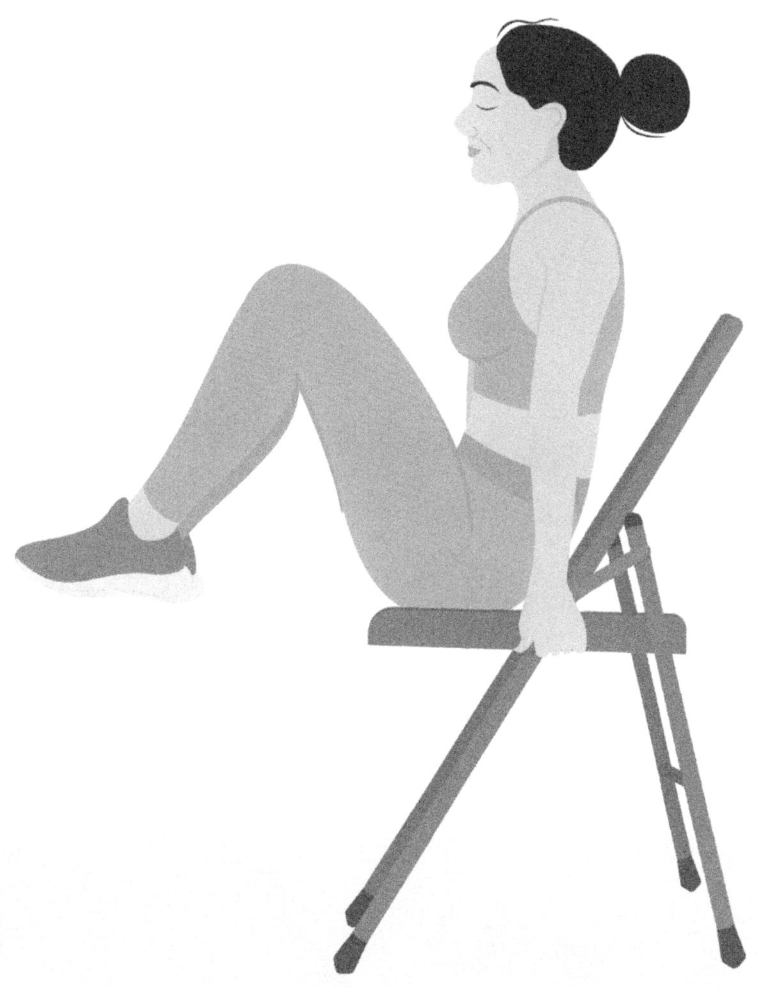

Elevation of the body

With this exercise you will be able to strengthen the abdomen and legs at the same time. To do this, you need to join your legs together while sitting in a chair.With your back straight, lift your knees towards your chest while keeping your abdomen taut. Now you will try to lift your body off the chair. Then, you will return to the starting position. Repeat this procedure 10 to 20 times.

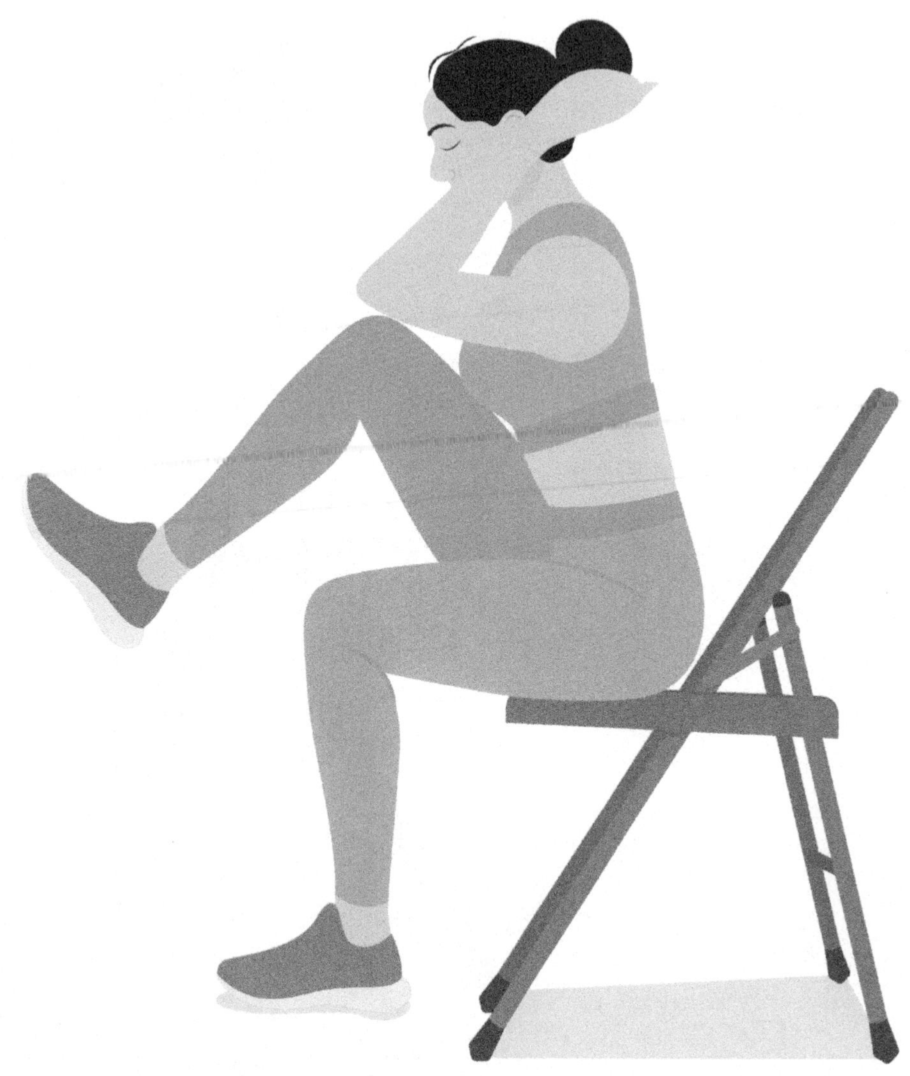

Knee towards the elbow

Thanks to this exercise you can work the lateral muscles and the abdominal area.To do this, sit in a chair with a straight back. Now, without leaning back, put your hands behind your neck. Now raise your right knee and touch it with your left elbow. Then, return to the starting position. Do 4 sets repeating 15 times with each side.

CHAPTER 15 EXERCISES TO LOSE WEIGHT TO DO IN BED

Is it really possible to practice Yoga anywhere? Maybe noteverywhere but in many more places than we think.

This is not an invitation not to get out of bed to practice, but I am sure you too have had a hell of a day and not been able to do your practice, and maybe now that it is evening you feel your back is in pieces and your body can't take it anymore.

When you are lying in bed before falling asleep, instead of checking your cell phone, you could do one, or more than one, of these positions to stretch and give your muscles some respite and relieve some stress.

They are all Asanas that are normally done on the mat, sitting orlying down and therefore fit perfectly to be practiced on the bed.

The Puppy Pose

The Puppy Pose is a mix of the Child Pose and the Downward Looking Dog Pose.

It's a great way to relax your body and stretch your back, back muscles, and increase shoulder mobility.

HOW YOU DO IT

From a four-legged position walk forward with your hands until you extend yourarms in front of you without moving the pelvis which remains stationary above the knees. Once you have reached the maximum stretch, gently push the chest down, opening the shoulders well and closing the shoulder blades. Make sure your shoulders are away from your ears.

Breathe deeply while continuing to seek the maximum reach.

The problem with this position is usually the knees that after a while on the hard floor begin to hurt, but on your bed this problem is avoided.

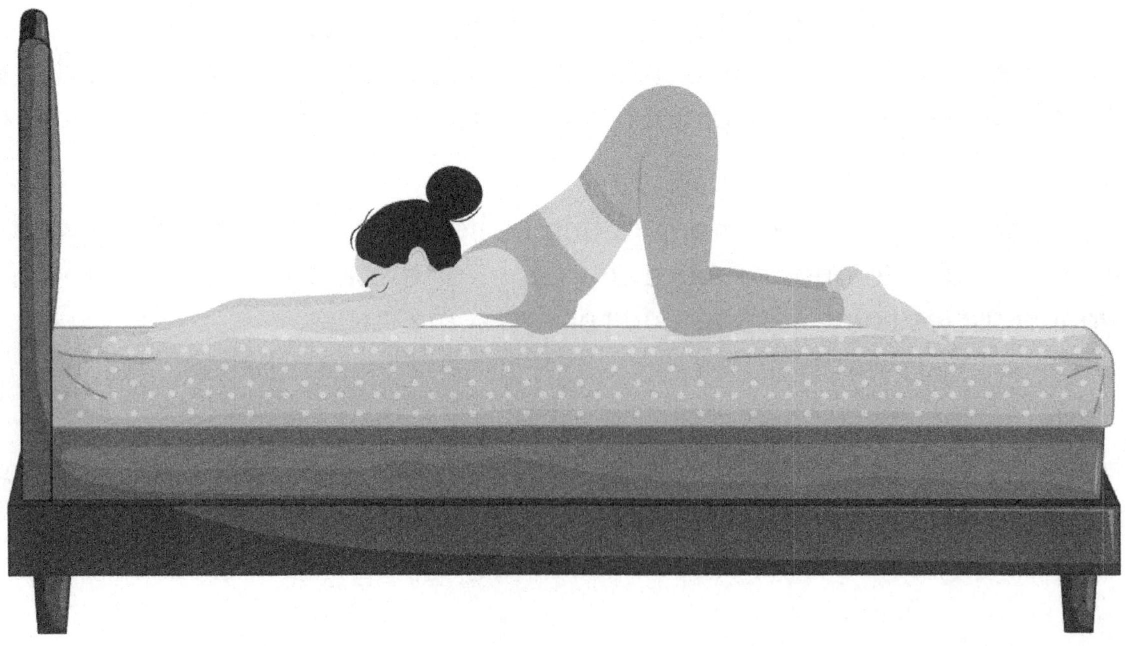

Puppy twist

It has all the benefits of the previous pose with the addition of twisting the spine, a great way to increase the hydration of your intervertebral discs subjected to being crushed all day and therefore a cure-all for the back.

How you do it

Also called the needle pose because you put your arm under your chest.

The position remains in all respects the same as the previous one with the difference that you try to rest your shoulder on the bed and turn your chest

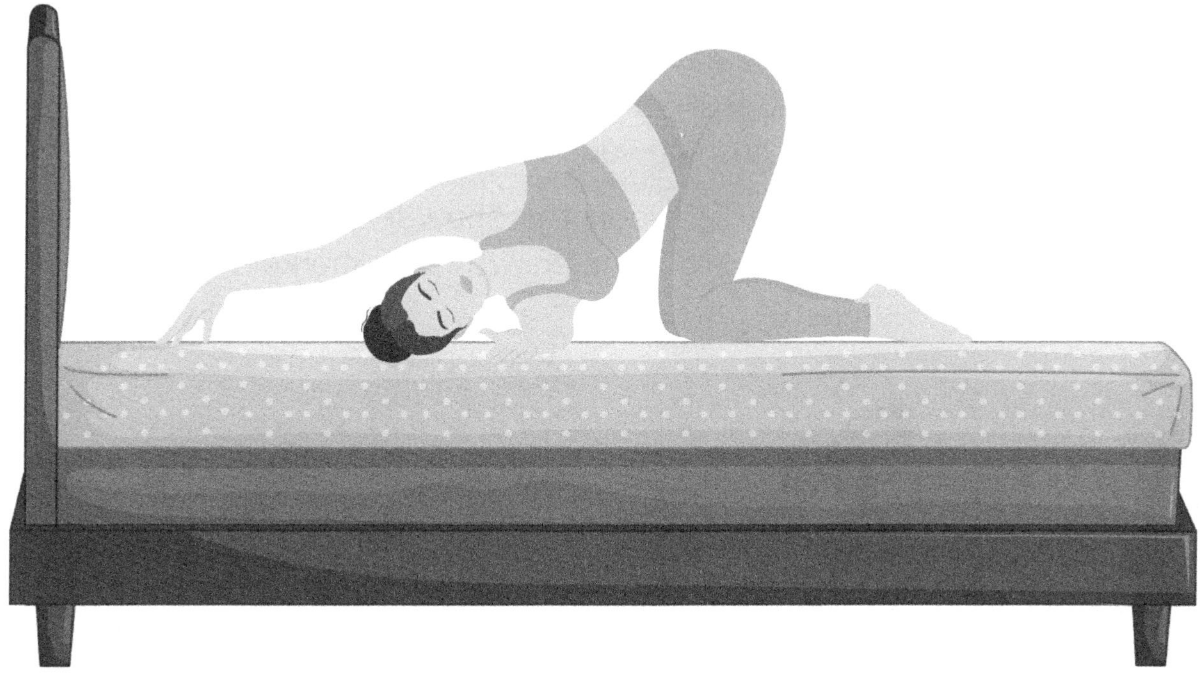

as much as possible towards the direction in which you brought your hand.

Breathing out, put your right arm under your chest, extending it to the left andattempting to lay your shoulder on the bed.

If you are unable to lean on the shoulder on the bed it is not a problem but you must still seek the maximum opening of the chest to the left, bringing the face as much as possible under the right armpit.

It should be done on both sides.

Sphinx

It is the simplified version of the "Cobra - Bhujangasana", but even if less intense,it is an excellent pose. Indeed, for some it is better than the complete one, to help loosen the back and reduce pain and tension.

It also stretches the abdominal muscles, increases the opening of the shoulders and chest, strengthens the shoulders.

HOW YOU DO IT

Lie on your stomach.

Keeping your elbows glued to the rib cage and maintaining good pressure on yourhands, lift your torso by pushing your shoulders down firmly.

The neck should not be sunk between the shoulders, if this happens it is becauseyou are not pushing hard enough with the shoulders down on the elbows.

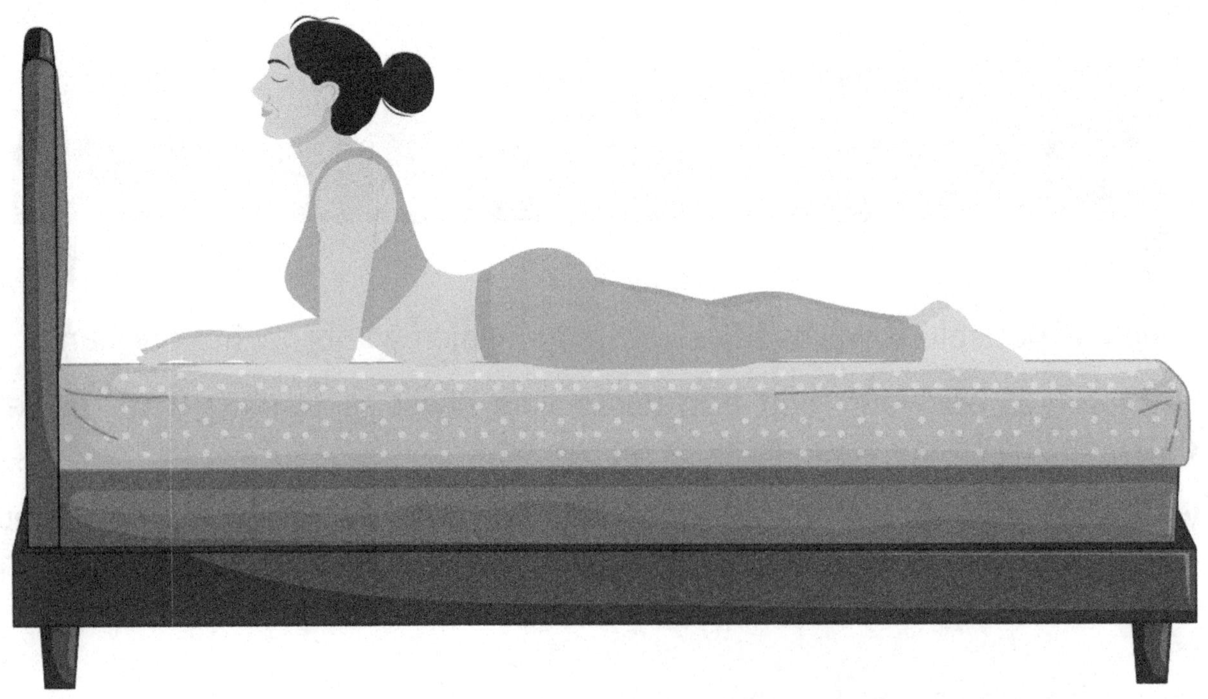

Elongated pigeon

This version, however, is more suitable for relaxing and stretching without major preparations. In this position, the psoas and rectus femoris hip flexors are stretched; it increases the opening of the inguinal muscles, the buttocks, relieving the tensionof the sciatic nerve and chronic back pain.

HOW YOU DO IT

Starting from a position where you are sitting on your heels, stretch your right leg back, moving your right foot as far away as possible from the left knee. The tibia is rotated until the left heel is aligned with the right hip.

Walking forward with your hands, you stretch as far forward as possible and once you have found the maximum extension, you relax on the leg that is bent.

If your hips are very closed it is possible that you will not succeed in the position, with the result that the body shifts to the side by placing one buttock on the bed, in this case the left.

By aligning the foot and the left knee the position is less intense and should be doable by everyone.

The pose is then repeated on the opposite side.

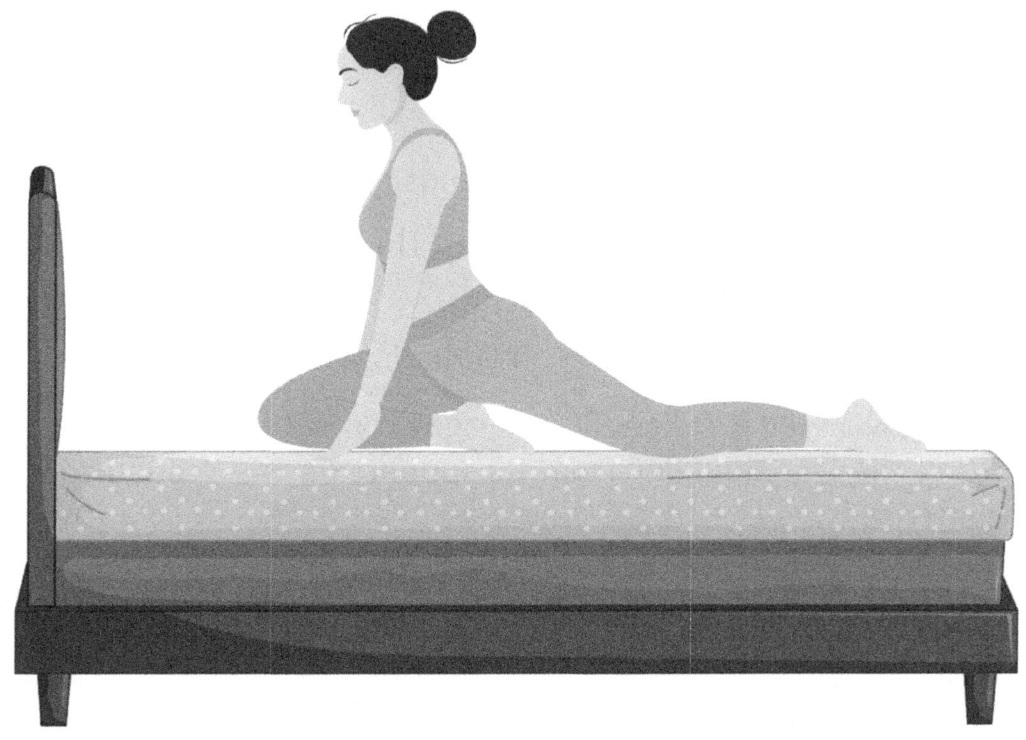

Supine torsion

This Asana is named after the Lord of fish, Matsyendra, who was a yogi and apupil of the god Shiva.

It is a truly relaxing and regenerating pose, suitable for everyone. Twists, ingeneral, are great for a healthy spine and healthy abdominal organs.

The supine twist helps the digestive system by massaging the colon and digestivetract.

It stretches the back muscles, stretches the buttocks and reduces tension in theshoulders, a place where they usually build up during the day.

How you do it

It starts from a lying position on your back. Feel that your whole back is well supported.

It is unlikely that the lower back is detached on a soft surface such as that of thebed, but if you do it on the ground and it should rise, gently press the lower parttowards the floor.

Open your arms in a cross, aligning your hands at shoulder height.

The right leg is fully extended, checking that the hip, knee and foot are in the same line.

Place the left foot on the right knee, thus flexing the left leg.

Go down gently with the left knee to the right trying to place it on the ground without lifting the left shoulder from its support on the ground to make the twistmore intense.

Repeat on the opposite side.

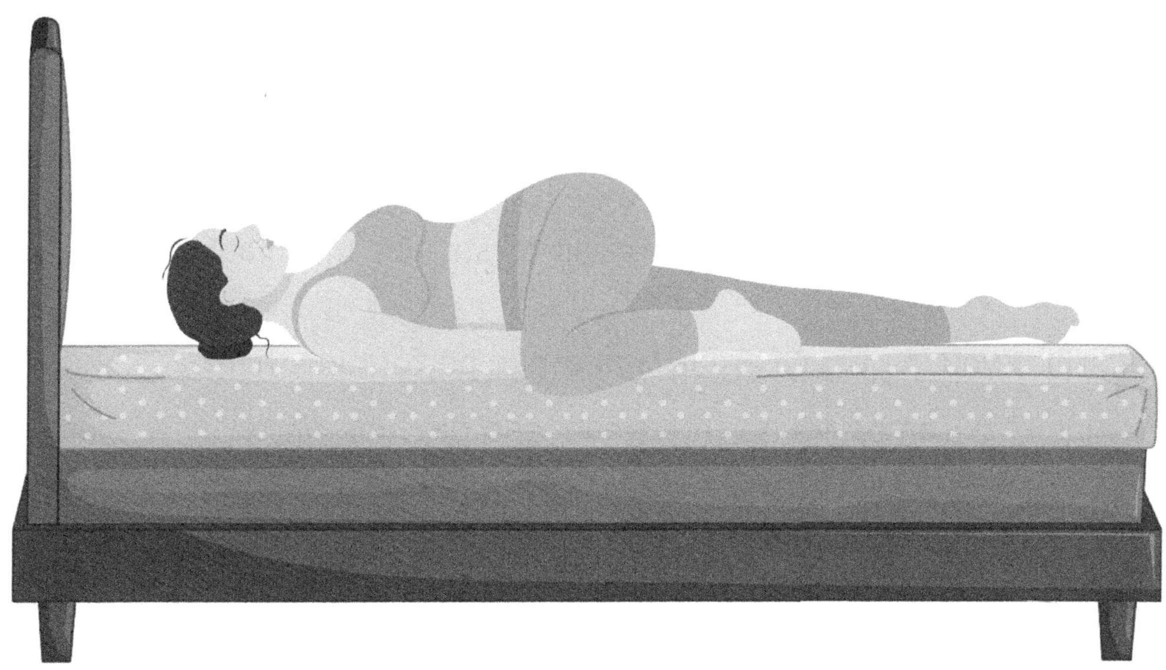

Relax first of all

These are all excellent positions to give respite to legs and back, tired from theworking day.

Above all, however, they are all very relaxing positions, so regardless of the intensity of your pose try to center your being on your breath, deep, carried downwards, towards the belly in order to stretch the diaphragm well, to maximize the relaxing experience.

Better still if you use Ujjayi pranayama while performing them.

Yoga moments can be found throughout the day, no matter how short they maybe.

Every moment "stolen" from the harmful habits to be given to the practice of Yoga brings great advantages over time both on a physical and psychological level.

CHAPTER 16 TIPS FOR YOGA PRACTICE AT HOME

Whether you attend a class in a yoga studio with a teacher, or if you want to tryfor the first time to approach this discipline on your own, when we decide to practice at home there is a moment of doubt: how to do yoga at home from alone?

Where to start individual practice?What to do if you are a beginner? Which exercises to choose?

DON'T THINK OF HAVING TO DO AT HOME WHAT YOU DID IN THE GROUP CLASS

Imagine the difference between a group lesson with a teacher and personal practice at home as the difference between eating in a restaurant or eating at home. You wouldn't judge your kitchen by comparing it to the restaurant's, right?

MAKE THE PRACTICE SHORT AND ENJOYABLE

A group class usually lasts from 60 to 90 minutes. If you start with this goal, it iseasy to give up quickly. Better to aim for a constant 10-15 min practice. Think of it like this: is it better to brush your teeth every day for a few minutes or go to the dentist once a month for an hour and a half?

CHOOSE A QUIET CORNER OF THE HOUSE AND CUSTOMIZE IT

If you are lucky enough to have a dedicated space, personalize it with candles, plants, incense, colored fabrics, music ... anything that can make it comfortableand to your liking. Do you only have a little space? Move some furniture, or use the balcony if you have one available. You can do the relaxation on the bed, thestanding positions or sitting on a chair. Get creative with the space available! Use the objects and furniture around you as supports.

START WITH WHAT YOU LIKE

If you have never tried yoga at home, it is best to start with the asanas and movements that you like the most and that you remember best, so as to also limit the risk of injury.

BE FLEXIBLE WITH THE TIMETABLE

The best time to practice is the one that best suits the schedule of your day andyour level of physical fatigue. For some it is better in the morning, for others itis better in the evening, for still others the quietest time available may be duringthe day. There is no rule: it is YOUR practice and you can change according to your needs.

BE FLEXIBLE WITH THE INTENSITY

The intensity of the practice must also be modulated around your needs. There will be days when you are more tired and days when you feel the need to discharge energy with more intense practice. The value of a personal practice isseen in the ability to tune in to your needs and respond appropriately.

TURN OFF THAT PHONE!

Most important of all, what makes yoga really effective, is that it is a moment of both mental and physical awareness. If we are continually distracted, we willnot get any results and it will be difficult to maintain the motivation to continue.

Let's start with a very simple practice that is performed by placing a chair in thesacred space you have chosen in the house.

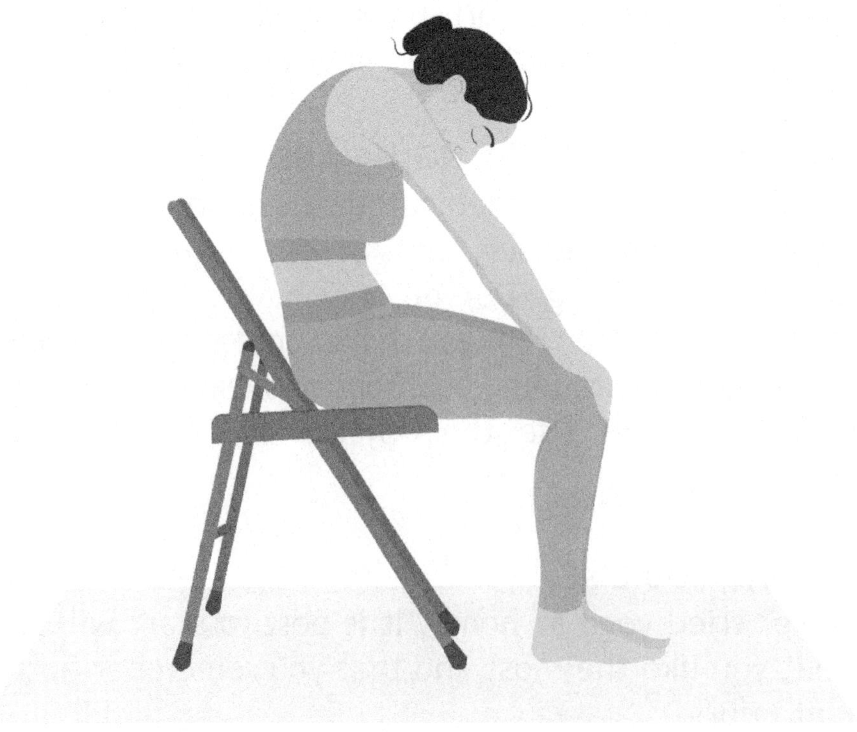

Start sitting on a chair to perform the spinal flexion exercise.

Initially you will send air to the lungs and diaphragm slowly and gently by inhalingthrough the nostrils.

If your nose is blocked, you can use your mouth.Inhalation will be done by

opening the chest.

After completing the deep inhalation, exhale bringing the navel inwards andemptying the diaphragm and lungs.

The chest movement will tilt the spine forward closing the chest and squeezingthe shoulders.

This exercise you will do repeatedly, for 2 to 3 minutes.

The spine is the area of the body that allows the natural mobility of our extremities and in turn allows the stability and firmness of our body.

In the past, a person's age was not calculated based on the years of life completed. But for the flexibility that the backbone showed.

This yoga exercise at home allows you to exercise spinal flexions and bring oxygen to the membranes of the spine, favoring the lower back, muscles and bones.

You will see that after resting and repeating the exercise, you can be more flexible on the second occasion you exercise. Which demonstrates the immediatebenefit of this exercise.

Once you have rested for about 30 seconds from the first exercise, I invite you to raise your arms in a deep inhalation and do a twist on the right side.

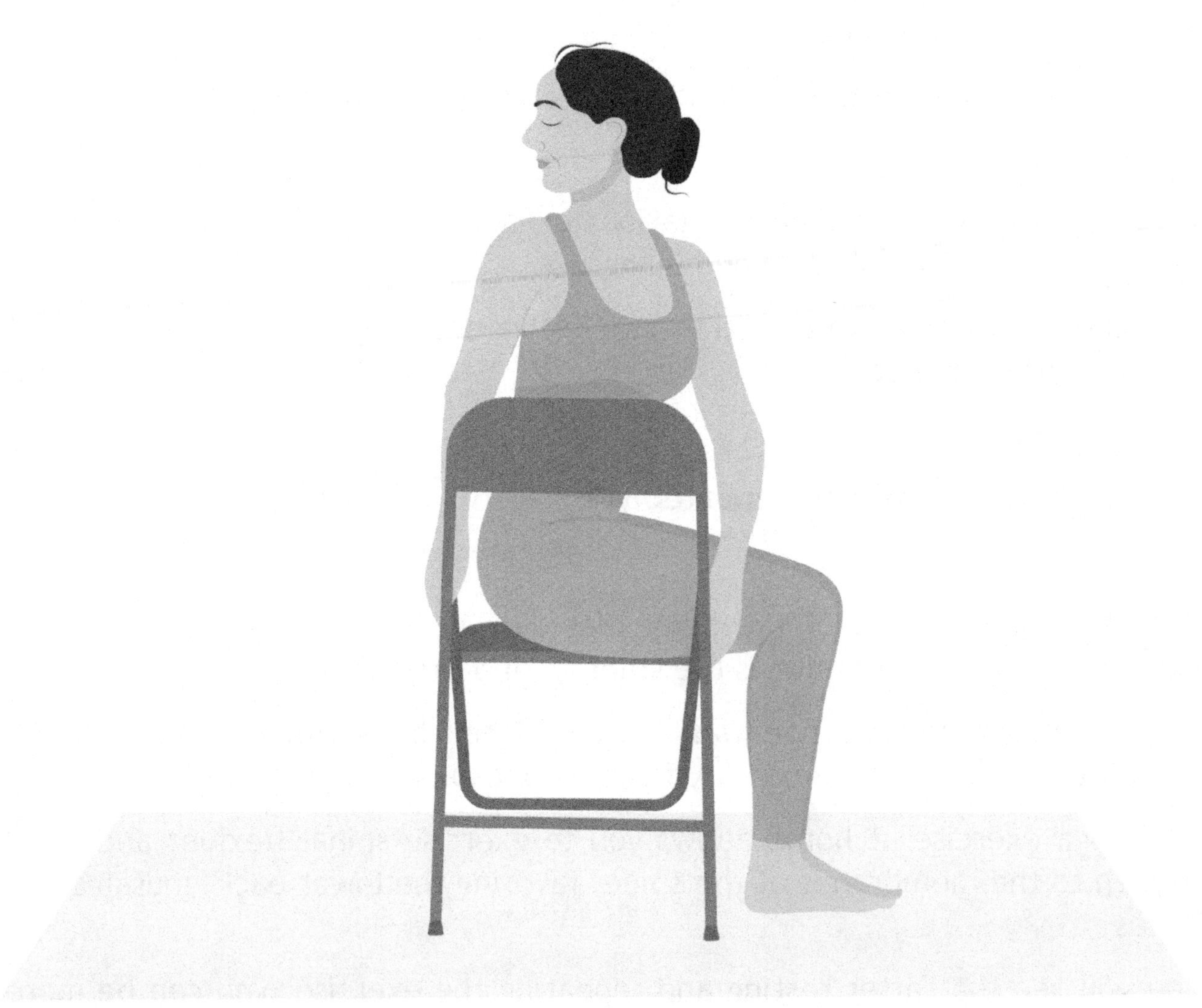

Help yourself by taking one side of the chair and bringing your left hand to yourright knee.

Try to bring your gaze to your right shoulder by doing a deeper twist. Remember to practice slow, natural and deep breathing during exercise.Take a minute to breathe and then slowly turn towards the center.

While sitting in the center, take 15 seconds of deep breathing and work your wayto the left side (opposite side) with the same twist.

Repeat the exercise in the same way and deepen your breathing.

Finish by returning to center and perform 15 seconds of deep breathing.

The deep breath is a breath that is described as a thread of light or Prana (vitalair) that penetrates our nostrils and that travels through our pharyngeal duct through our chest, filling our diaphragm like a bomb and filling our lungs withoutforcing. That is done at 2-3 second intervals.

This breath leads us to feel the beating of our heart and our blood system. Activating our vision and extra sensory sense.

Raise your arms in a powerful inhalationStay seated.

Once you have raised your arms in a powerful inhalation, exhaleand bring your hands to the ground with your legs half open.

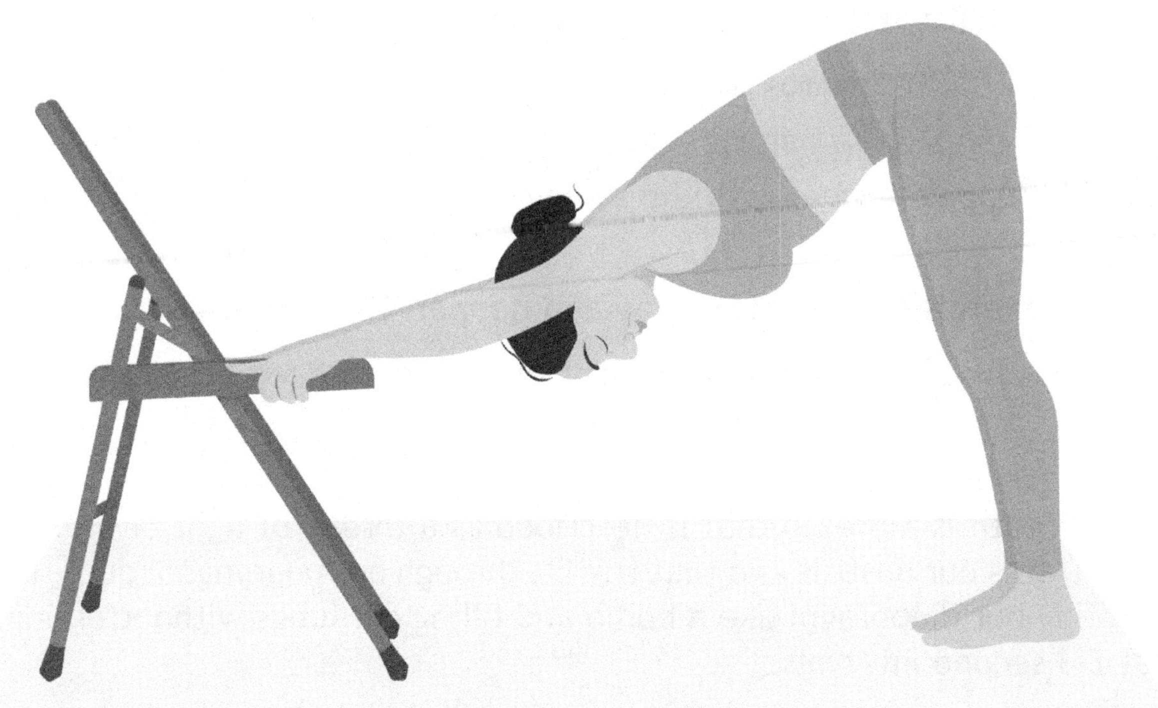

Rest your back.

Relax your arms, shoulder blades and trapezius.

Drop the weight of your head by relaxing your neck.

Breathe fully and deeply for 1-2 minutes.

The force of light

By performing these exercises, you will activate your magneticfield and your immune system. Tranquility in motion is the activation of our light and extrasensory field. This allows us to protect ourselves through the force of light like a mirror that repels negative force.

Go back to the center and stand up. Stand in front of the center of your chair.Inhale and raise your arms in a V shape.

Exhale out of the nose by lowering the trunk and hands towards the chair.

Put your hands on the seat and let the weight of your head drop.

Bend your elbows and rest the forehead on the connected arms to rest your entiretorso and back.

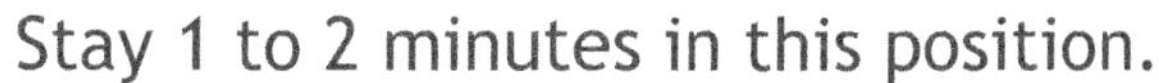

Stay 1 to 2 minutes in this position.

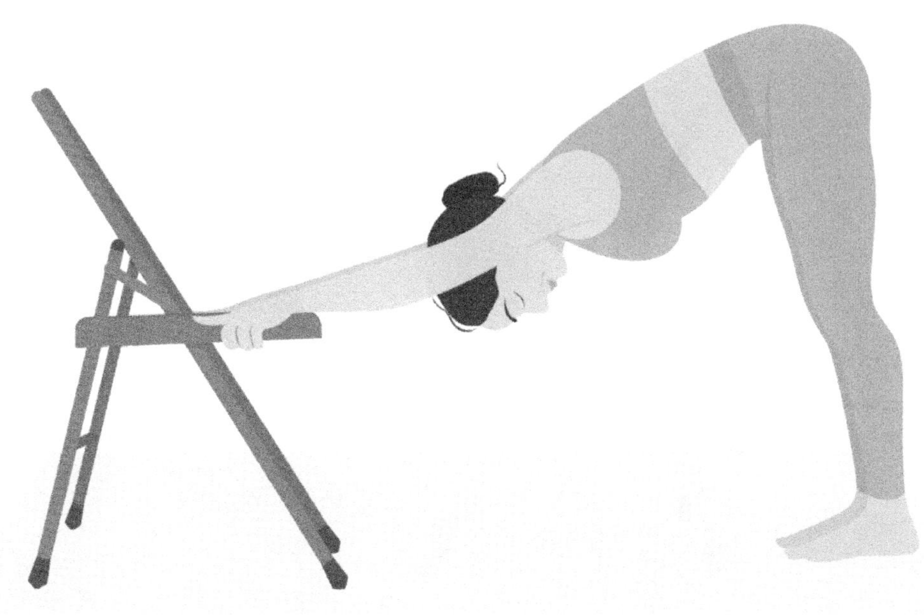

Neck and middle back

This position is very special for those who suffer from pain in the neck and middleback.

Bring your legs to the seat of your chair by flexing your knee.Bring your hands to your chest and feel your breath.

Relax your jaw and facial muscles.

Focus on a straight position, resting the base from the legs.Breathe for 3 minutes.

Return with a stronger breath to get out of the position and wake up.Now remove the chair and stretch your legs on the floor.

Bring your arms to the sides of your body with your palms facing the sky.

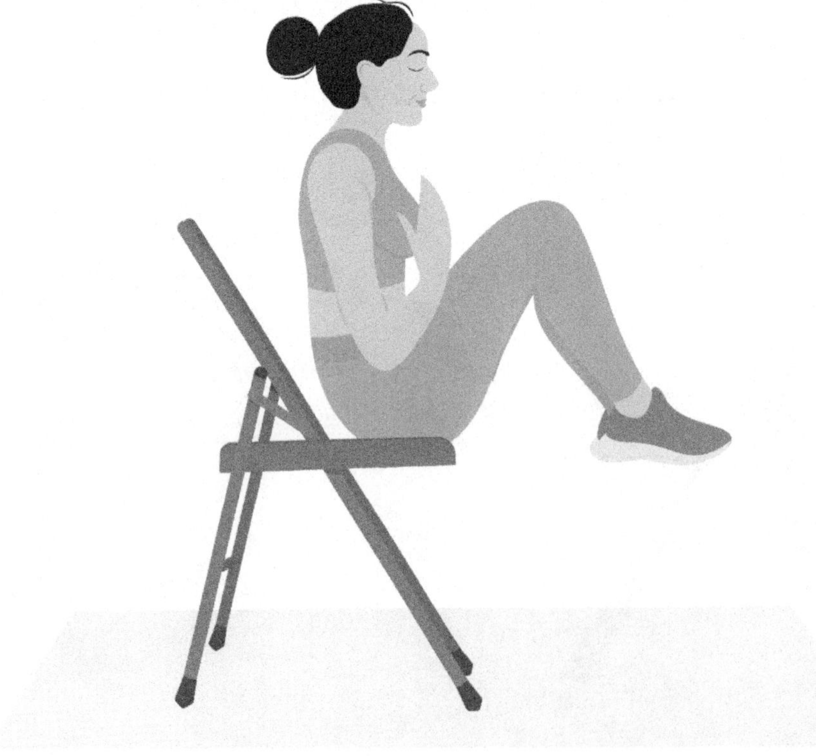

Relax in this variation of the Savasana posture or corpse posture.Release all tension and weight.

During this session, try to dedicate yourself to yourself and check your blocks ineach exercise in order to always be able to flow better within your yoga exercisesat home.

Always trust in yourself, in the divinity that is your pure soul, that power that guides you to advance in everything that you propose to yourself.

Your magnetic field will be strengthened and you will attract forces that will allow you to integrate and be in harmony with the whole.

Your cellular memory will be it will be in constant motion, you will strengthen the positive elements of your memories and you will remove blocks and structures that prevent you from advancing into other phases of your life.

All of this can be done through this type of practice in which conscious breathingand movement are included while respecting your personal field.

Appreciate your line of consciousness to achieve your life purpose in full realization.

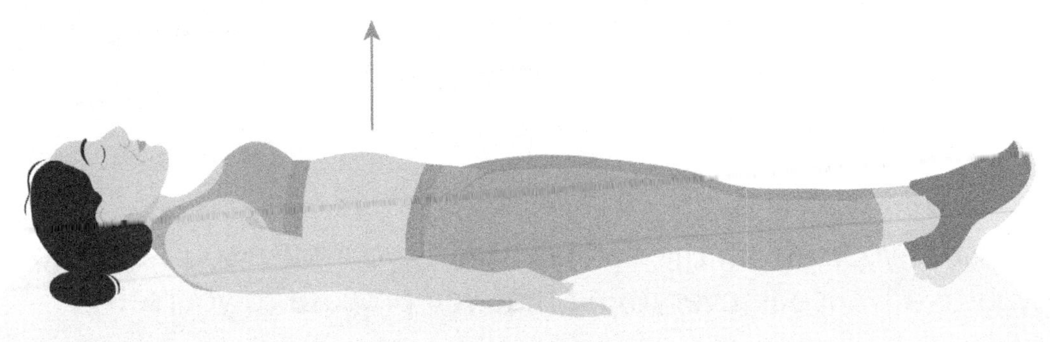

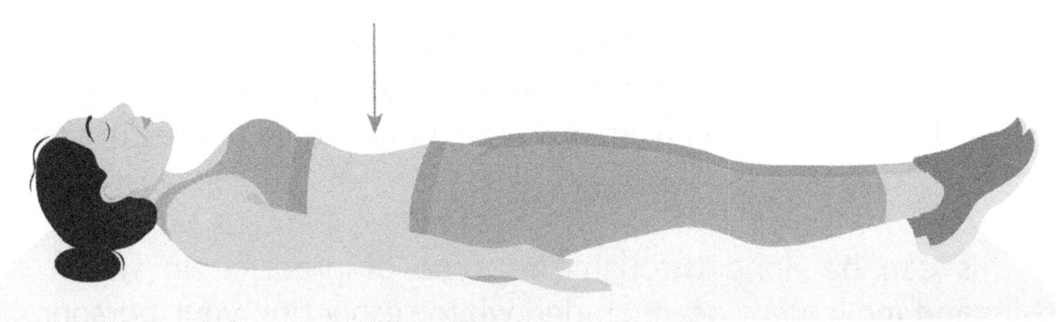

CHAPTER 17 THE IMPORTANCE OF THE BREATH

Breathing is one of the foundations of yoga, along with meditation and the practice of physical exercises, asanas. The three practices are to be understoodas inseparable, because only from their union is it possible to fortify the body and free the mind by elevating the spirit. Yoga introduces the importance of breathing through a fundamental concept, namely the knowledge of its vital function. Man can, in fact, go a few days without food, but he can never stop breathing. In light of this concept, breathing is considered as a fundamental partof the discipline, as an art who asks to be cultivated with targeted breathing exercises capable of calming the mind, observing and controlling the breath to shape it according to one's needs.

Unfortunately, modern man has forgotten how he breathes and does it very oftenin the wrong way, filling the belly with useless air and therefore not regeneratingthe cells that make up the body. The result is a series of ailments that can be effectively combated with the right yogic breathing. Let us remember that the influx of oxygen to the brain is obtained through breathing, so by implementinga correct practice, the mind is allowed to function in a more lucid and active way, as well as to face problematic moments with better safety and with vigorousinner strength.

The purpose of yoga breathing exercises is mainly to fill the lungs with fresh air,starting from the lower abdomen to reach the upper airways such as the nose and throat. To implement this technique, yoga relies on pranayama, or exercises that are introduced together with the practice of asanas, or performed independently and linked to the meditative process.

Breathing is living, but we don't always remember it. We do it automatically, almost always badly, without filling and emptying the lungs adequately.

It is said that good breathing is the basis of the psycho-physical balance of everyhuman being. What is certain is that the yoga discipline, in particular Hatha, alsocalled yoga of longevity, attributes central importance to the breathing techniques to be applied during the execution of the exercises, or the asanas. Ifyou think about it, it is not surprising.

Have you noticed how many times, when you are under stress, anxious or very focused on something, you literally forget to breathe? Stay in apnea? For 10, 20,30 seconds? A lack of oxygenation not compensated by an adequate inflow of airto the lungs in the following inspirations, usually short and shallow.

Nobody teaches us to breathe. It is a natural act, just like eating, walking, talking. Indeed, the rhythmic act of inhaling and exhaling is the first sign of life(and of a healthy and robust constitution), of the newborn emerging from the maternal womb after birth.

To breathe is to live. Simple.

For this reason, yoga, which is not just any gymnastics, but the sum of Indian wisdom applied to the body and mind, identifies precisely in breathing the actionthat binds the physical part to the psychic and spiritual part of human beings. Itteaches us to improve our health and to reach a state of balance and well-beingthanks to a well-balanced mix of meditation (to discipline the mind) and physicaltraining (to sculpt the body). In all of this, breathing well is essential.

It is not difficult; you just have to "think about it". Being present in the moment, aware of your body in every fiber, without any distractions, without interference. Here are some basic yoga breathing techniques, of which the firsttwo - abdominal and thoracic breathing - are the most important, to learn whichyou need a quiet environment, solitude, 15-20 minutes of your time, preferablyin the morning.

The ideal position to practice these techniques is to be lying down (on the mat or even on the bed). Alternatively, you can settle into standing with your hands on your hips, or sitting, with your torso erect and legs stretched out in front of you or crossed under you.

Abdominal breathing

Focus your mental attention on your belly.

Inhale slowly

and always slowly raise the abdomen, so that it is pushed - but without forcing -towards the chest.

When you have filled the stomach with air up to the diaphragm, release gentlyas you exhale.

Empty your lungs by lowering your abdomen as far as possible.

Repeat this breathing technique several times gently, calmly, until you go on automatic.

Duration: from a minimum of 2 minutes to a maximum of 5. You can use astopwatch for times.

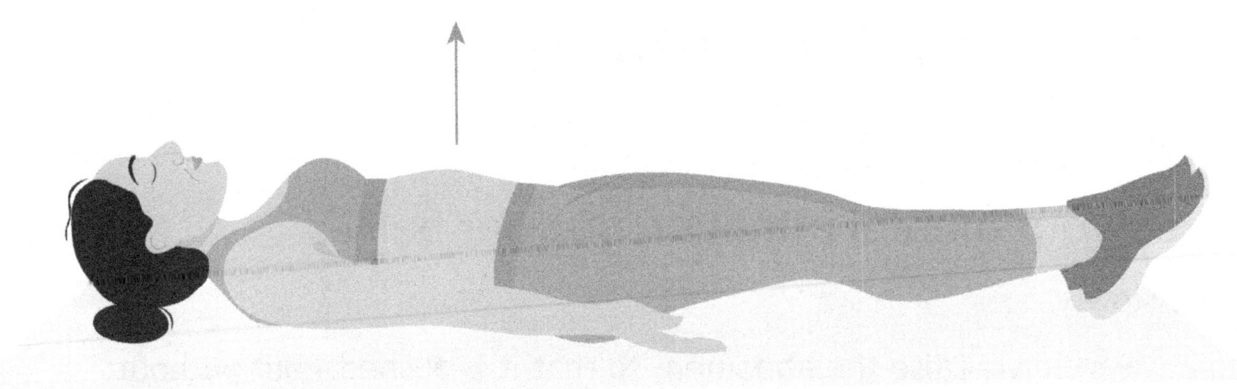

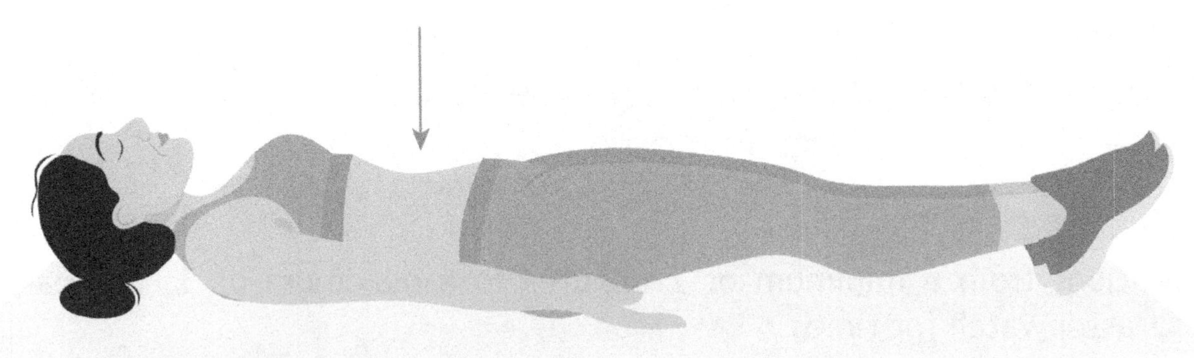

Thoracic breathing

Focus on the chest muscles and contract the pectoral muscles gently.

Breathe in slowly through your nose, but without using your belly in any way.

Instead, fill your chest with air as much as you can, right up to the "brim".

Then start releasing the air by exhaling for a long time,

slowly but completely, and this time you can lower your abdomen slightly.

Duration: from 2 to 5 minutes

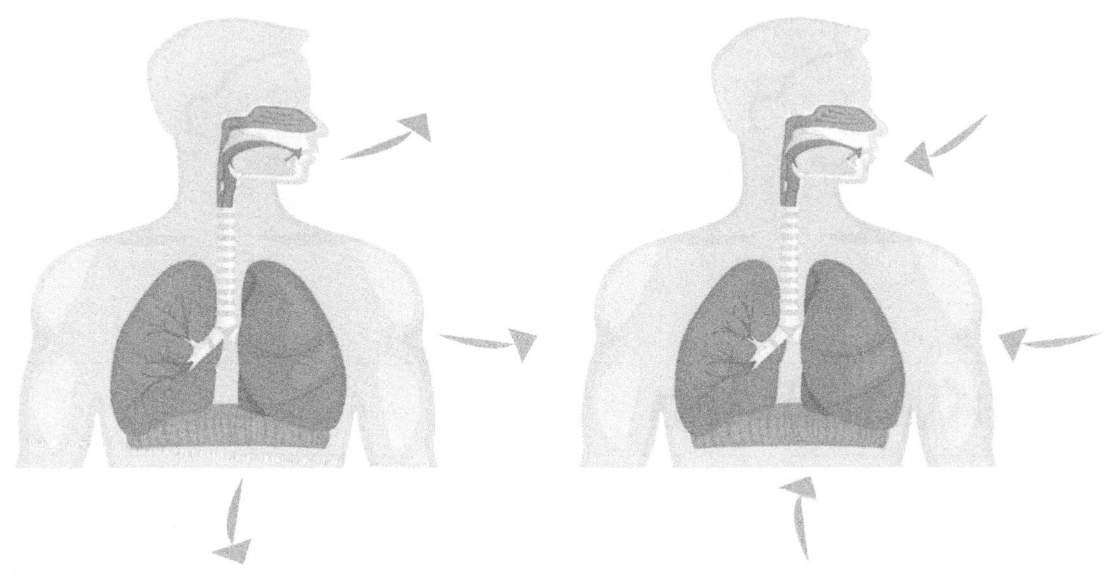

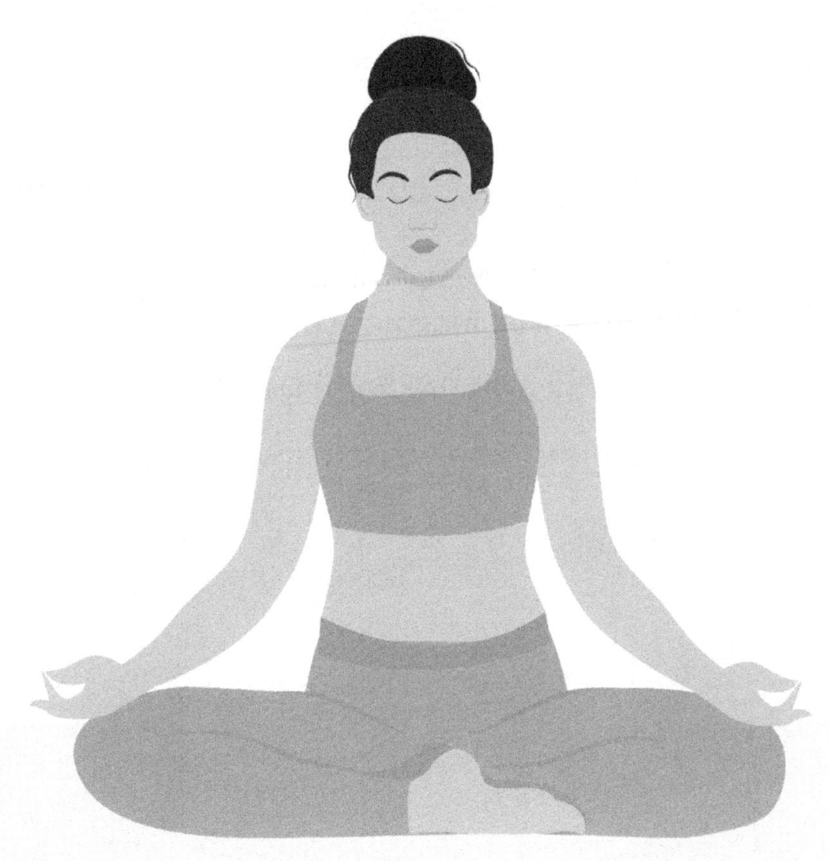

Kumbhaka

Kumbhaka is a basic yoga breathing exercise, which is performed by inspiring and counting up to eight seconds.

This is then followed by a retention of eight seconds and an exhalation of thesame duration. Students who become good at it can continue the exercise byincreasing the number of seconds, reaching a maximum of 32.

This yoga breathing exercise helps to calm nervous states, especially if prolonged, but it is never correct to strain as the increase in seconds must be carried out in proportion to one's physical possibilities.

The purifying breath serves, as the name suggests, to clean the lungs, especially after staying in poorly ventilated and unhealthy places. It is one of thesimplest and most immediate yoga breathing exercises to implement, as it is sufficient to inhale slowly through the nose and then exhale immediately by parting the lips and then expelling the air strongly and quickly through the mouth. This yoga breathing exercise can be repeated several times a day, as needed.

One of the most important aspects of yoga practice is Pranayama, or the science related to the study of breath.

And one of the most important is what is called "the breath of fire", its name in Sanskrit is Agni Pran.

This breathing technique is so called because it has a direct action on our belly, on our inner fire and on the energy point it guards called the "third chakra", and it is precisely this point to which the fire element is connected.

The basic pump movement that characterizes it is focused precisely in thediaphragm area.

This breath can be practiced alone, but it is also often found in sequences,combined with certain positions or movements, and in many meditations.

WHAT'S IT ABOUT?

The breath of fire is rapid and vigorous abdominal breathing, generally done fromthe nose but in some cases, when specified, it also occurs from the mouth.

The inhalation and exhalation are equal in duration and intensity, there is no pause between them and the rhythm is fast with about 2 or 3 breaths per second.

Our attention must be focused especially on exhalation, every time the air quickly leaves the nose, the diaphragmatic area, that is the area from the navelupwards, retracts backwards and upwards, towards the column, making the air exit the lungs. The next inhalation will be a consequent relaxation of the area just contracted, without forcing the movement, the belly will go out by reflex. It is a movement that becomes automatic with practice if you focus on the contraction of the belly on the exhale.

Until we are very familiar with this breathing, it is advisable to keep a slower rhythm, in order to feel the right movement of the diaphragm well, and as you become familiar you will be able to maintain the right rhythm.

My suggestion is to always start with short cycles of 10/15 breaths of fire interspersed with a few deep breaths.

Begin practicing the Breath of Fire

Normally this pranayama is used within a sequence or meditation, but it can stillbe practiced individually, sitting in one of the various meditative positions, for example Sukhasana or easy position, Padmasana or the lotus position, Vajrasana,or the position of the rock.

Sitting on a chair with the soles of the feet in contact with the floor or lying on the ground, they are two very easy positions to learn to recognize diaphragmaticbreathing and to train with the breath of fire.

It is important to keep the spine straight with a slight closing of the chin towardsthe chest.

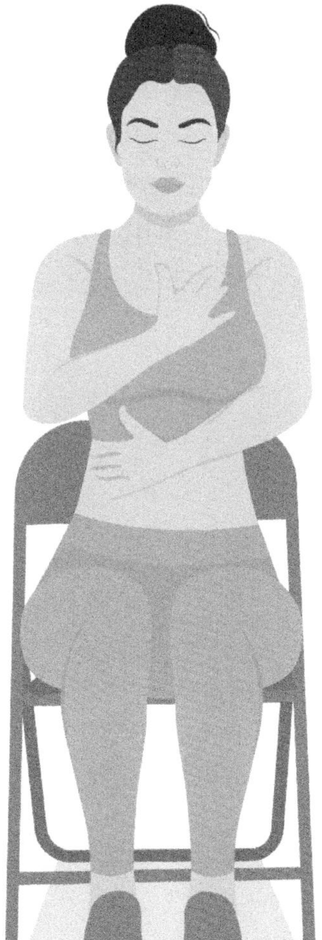

The hands can be in the prayer mudra, on the knees joining index and thumb inGyan Mudra or in the lap with the palms facing up.

To start, it is very useful to put your hands on the belly to observe the movementof the belly and to help with a very light pressure on the navel to facilitate exhalation.

The chest remains relaxed and slightly raised throughout the breath cycle.

Some people breathe paradoxically and this means that they will tend to do theopposite movement: in the exhalation there will not be a push towards the column of the diaphragmatic area but towards the outside. Usually when you arein this situation, you cannot produce a well-done breath of fire and it takes a lotof effort. The best thing to do is to do it very slowly, trying to consciously reverse the thrusting movement of the belly, or to become familiar with this pump movement and practice it without pairing the breath for a few minutes and thenstart combining the breathing calmly, always taking the time to stop breathing normally and then try again.

It is good to start the practice of the breath of fire calmly and take the time to strengthen and train the muscles of the abdominal wall and around the navel, which we often do not have the habit of using.

Effects and benefits

The powerful pump movement that is created in the navel causes a strong concentration of prana in this area, favoring a strong energy recharge. The activation of the fire element sets in motion a purification process, which generally "burns" toxins throughout the body, both physical, energetic and psychic.

It may happen that your practice generates a sense of nausea and dizziness, all signs that toxins have been set in motion that the system is trying to eliminate.If this happens, it is good to drink a lot of water and eat in a light and vegetarianway to encourage the cleaning process that has been activated, even better if vegan.

Sit in one of the meditative positions, bring your hands in the prayer mudra to your chest, open first with the mantras of the Kundalini Yoga tradition.

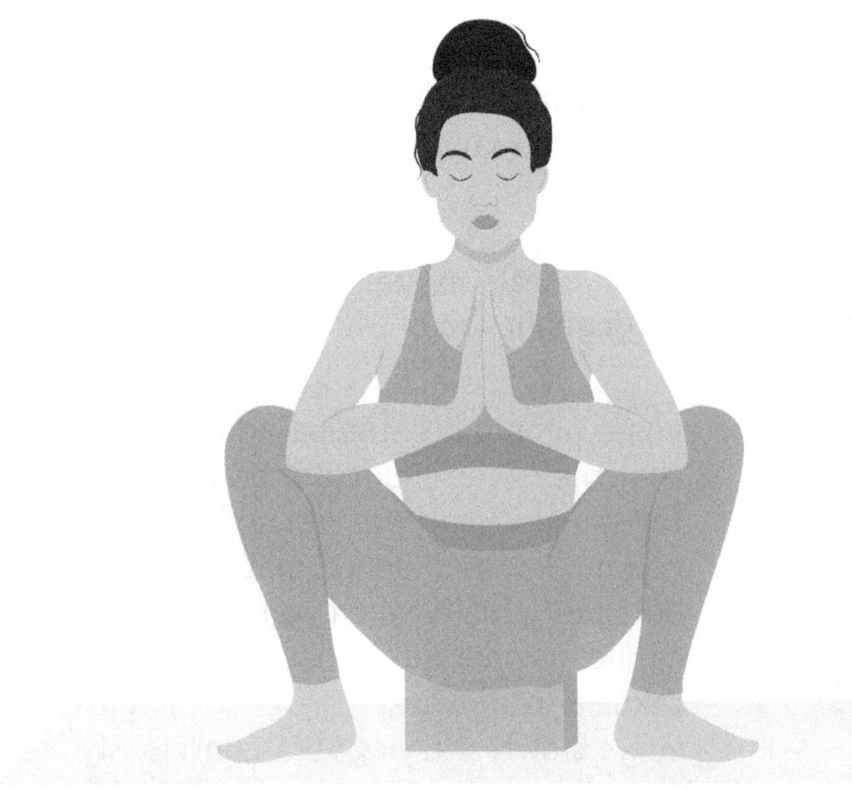

Basic combination, to be repeated 3 to 5 times:

Close the eyes nearly completely, turning the eyes up, towards the third eye.

If you have difficulty producing the movement, try to practice it without pairingit with your breath, for 1 to 3 minutes.

Practice the fire breath for 1 to 3 minutes

To close, inhale deeply through the nose, keep the air in for 10 seconds, alwaysexhale through the nose, and relax.

Remain in the position and bring your hands in Gyan Mudra on your knees, withyour arms outstretched and palms forward.

Observe the spontaneous flow of breath for 3 minutes.Inhale deeply, exhale.

Repeat the cycle if you want.

FINAL TIPS AND CONCLUSIONS

Losing weight with yoga is something really simple. It will not only change your body, but over time, your mind as well.

Since practicing yoga, food has ceased to be my obsession: before I stuffed myself with steaks and salads - at lunch and dinner - to stimulate the action of the muscles and prevent the accumulation of sugars in the body.

I only indulged in a piece of chocolate cake on Sundays and had practically forgotten the taste of pasta.

Yoga made me freer: I stopped gorging myself on protein and gladly accepted starches as well.

I no longer gained weight, also simply because I stopped thinking about how manycalories a plate of spaghetti has before piercing a forkful. It may seem trivial, but your mind does more than you think.

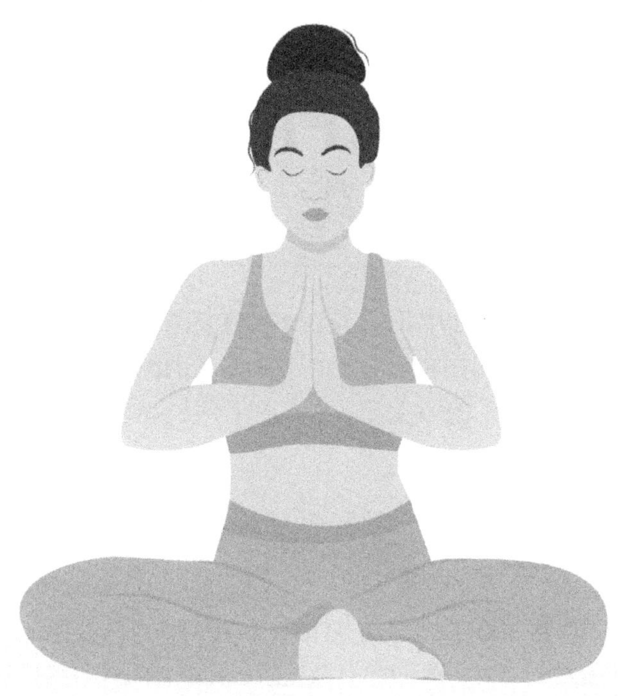

Utthita Parsvakonasana

It is a position that you can do either alone or with the help of a chair if you area beginner. This asana stimulates the thigh muscles and, being an open twist, also the abdominal band and hips. It is important that the weight is well distributed over the whole body. Beginners can sit on a chair with legs togetherand bring the right hand to the ground and the left hand to the sky. If possible, try to look up to the ceiling to increase the twist. Repeat on the other side.

Chair yoga classes can help improve flexibility and range of motion, as well as increase strength and endurance. Additionally, it can help reduce stress and anxiety levels. Chair yoga is also a great way to get some light exercise.

If you are unable to do more strenuous forms of yoga, all you need is to sit comfortably and have a sturdy chair. As with any exercise, if you have any existing health conditions, consult a medical professional before trying this exercise!

THE HEALTH BENEFITS OF CHAIR YOGA

This style of yoga can be done while sitting in a chair. It is ideal for those who have difficulty standing or balance problems. Chair yoga can also be done by people of all ages and fitness levels.

REVIEWED STUDIES INCLUDE:

Improved flexibility: it is no secret that one of the benefits of yoga is the improvement of flexibility. When we stretch our muscles, we not only increase our range of motion, but we also improve the elasticity of our muscles and connective tissues. This can lead to better posture and a reduced risk of injury.Not to mention that it feels good!

Increased strength: while increased flexibility is one of the best-known benefitsof yoga, increased strength is often overlooked. However, with regular practice,you can expect to see a significant increase in core muscles and endurance. Thisis especially beneficial for those who are unable to participate in more traditional forms of exercise.

Improved balance and coordination: yoga requires you to use your body in new and stimulating ways. This can help improve your balance and coordination, as well as your proprioception (your ability to feel where your body is in space). Improving these skills can help reduce the risk of falls and injuries.

Better Mind-Body Connection: one of the unique aspects of yoga is that it requires you to be fully present in the moment. This can help improve your mind-body connection or your awareness of your body and its movements. With regularpractice, you can learn to control your body with greater precision and ease.

Improved circulation: when practicing yoga, it helps pump oxygen-rich blood toall parts of the body, including organs and tissues. This can lead to better overallhealth and function. Plus, better circulation can help reduce pain and inflammation.

Better posture: by stretching your muscles, you can improve your alignment andlearn to stand (and sit) taller. This can help reduce pain and stiffness, as well asimprove your overall appearance.

Reduction in stress and anxiety levels: should come as no surprise that one of the main benefits of yoga is the reduction of stress and anxiety levels. When youpractice yoga, it helps to calm and relax your mind and body. This can lead to areduction in stress hormones, such as cortisol. Additionally, yoga can help increase serotonin and gamma- aminobutyric acid (GABA) levels, which are known to promote relaxation and calm. This will also help your sleep habits.

FOUR ESSENTIAL POSITIONS OF CHAIR YOGA

This practice is a great way to do yoga without having to go down onto the floor.Here is a complete guide to these four common chair yoga positions.

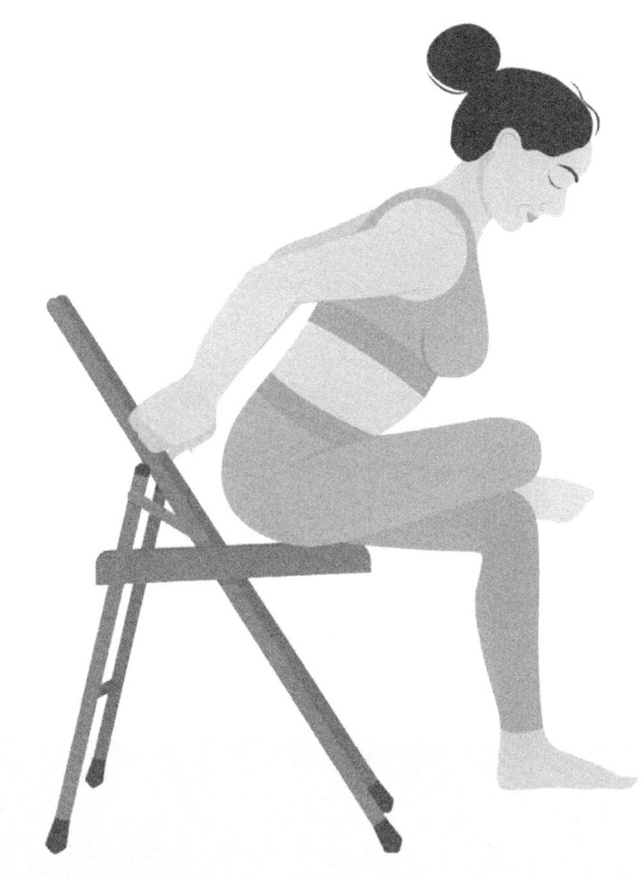

CHAIR EAGLE - GARUDASANA

To do Chair Eagle, start in a seated position with your feet flat on the ground and your hands resting in your lap. From there, lift your right leg and place yourright ankle over your left knee. Then, lean forward at the waist and stretch yourarms around the back of your chair. Hold on to the back of the chair with both hands and try to straighten up as much as you can. Maintain this position for 30 seconds to a minute before switching sides.

CHAIR FORWARD BEND - UTTANASANA

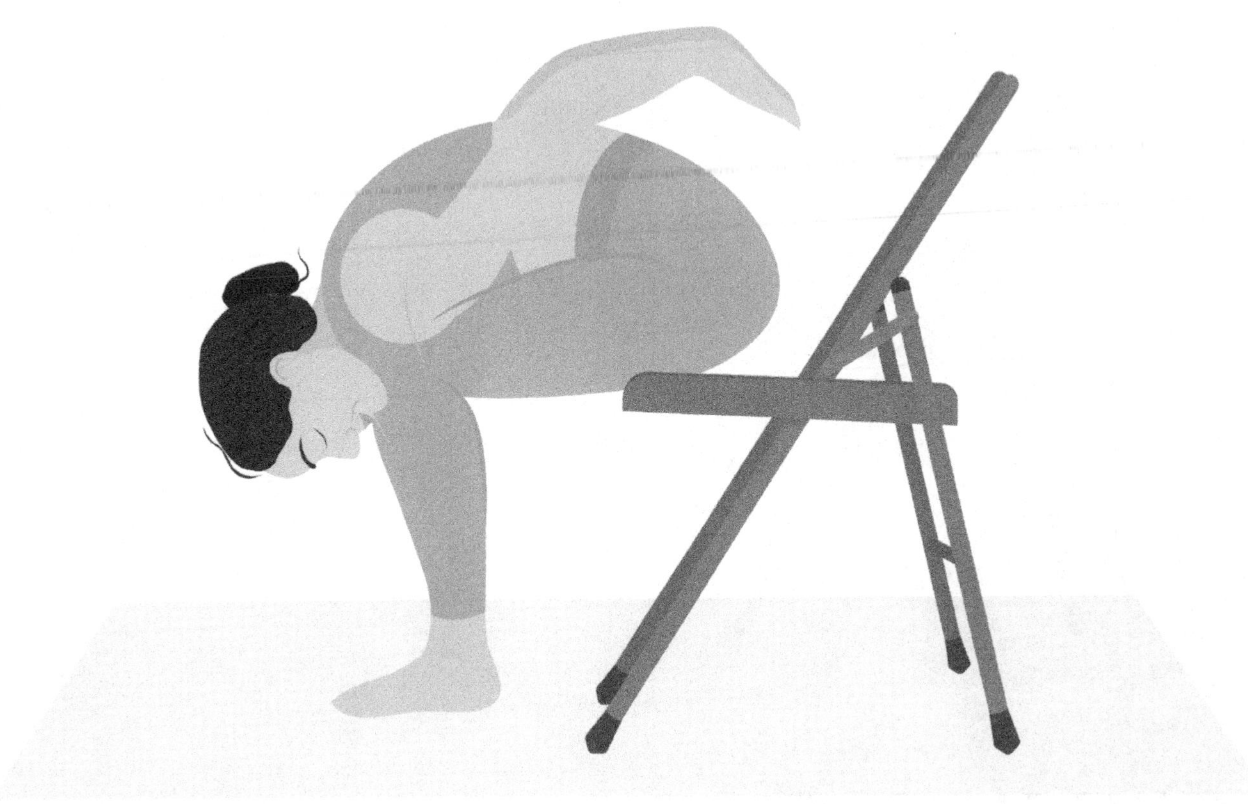

To do Chair Forward Bend, begin in a sitting position with your feet flat on the ground and your hands resting in your lap. From there, stretch your arms up and then lean forward from the waist, bringing your chest towards your thighs. Try to keep your back as straight as possible as you reach the ground with both hands. Maintain this position for 30 seconds toone minute.

SEATED MOUNTAIN (TADASANA)

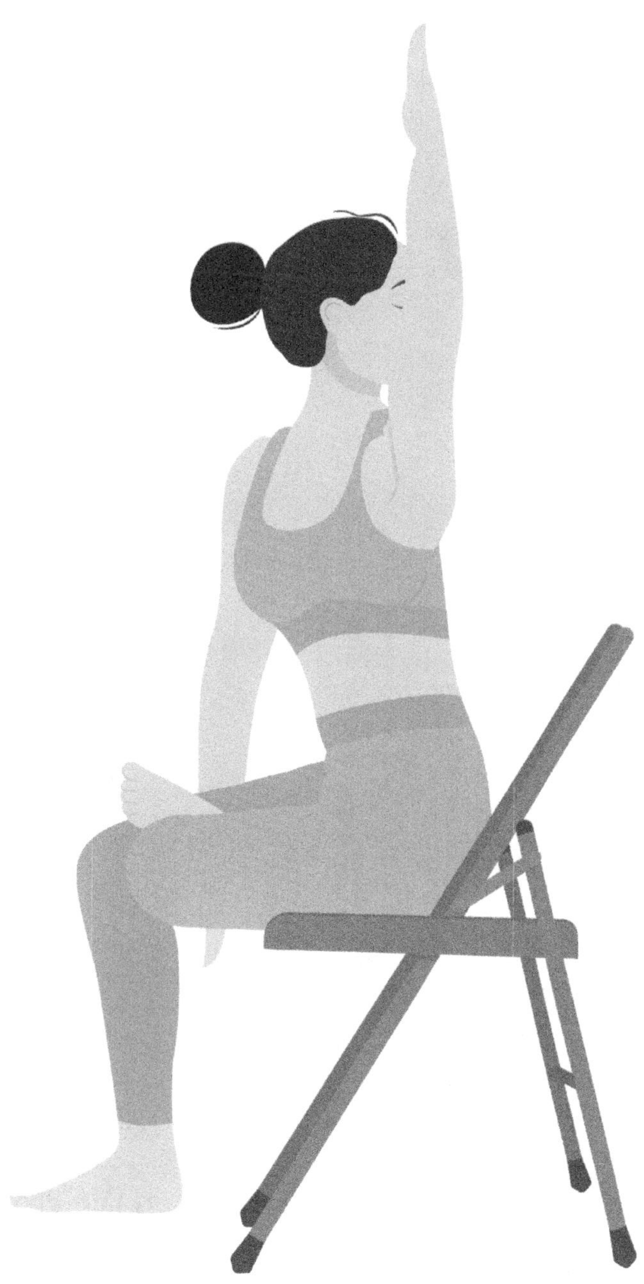

To do Seated Mountain, start in a seated position with your feet flat on the ground and your hands resting on your lap. From there, lift your right leg and place your right foot on the seat of the chair. Then, rotate the torso to the left,reaching the left arm up. Try to keep your back as straight as possible as you reach the ground with your right hand. Maintain this position for 30 seconds to aminute before switching sides.

EAGLE ARMS (GARUDASANA ARMS)

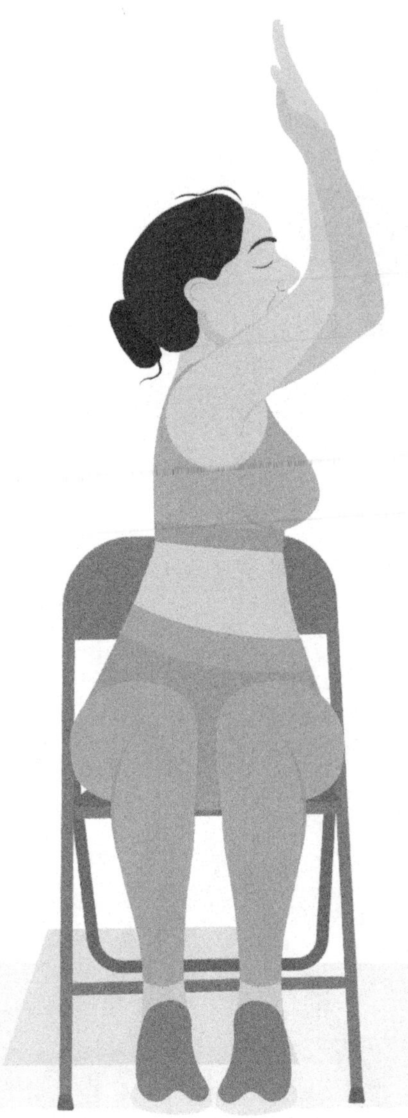

To do Eagle Arms, start in a seated position with your feet flat on the ground andyour hands resting in your lap. From there, raise your right arm and place your right elbow over your left elbow. Then, rotate your torso to the right, reaching your left arm behind your back. Try to keep your back as straight as possible as you reach the ground with your right hand. Maintain this position for 30 secondsto a minute before switching sides.

When you're done, return to a sitting position with your feet flat on the ground and your hands in your lap. Take several breaths and relax in this position for one minute.

So, there you are - some poses you can do anywhere, anytime! Try it because it'san easy but effective way to start the day or to break up a long day at work.

TWO BREATHING EXERCISES FOR CHAIR YOGA

When we think of yoga, we often think of people turning their bodies into pretzel-like shapes on a mat. However, yoga is much more than that. Yoga is a practice of the mind and body that includes breathing work, meditation and physical postures. While some people are able to do more advanced yoga poses,others need to modify the poses or use props such as chairs.

There are many different breathing exercises that can be done while sitting in achair. Here are two different exercises to try:

Dirga pranayama

The first of the two exercises, also known as the three-part breath.

This exercise helps calm the nervous system and is a great way to start practicing.

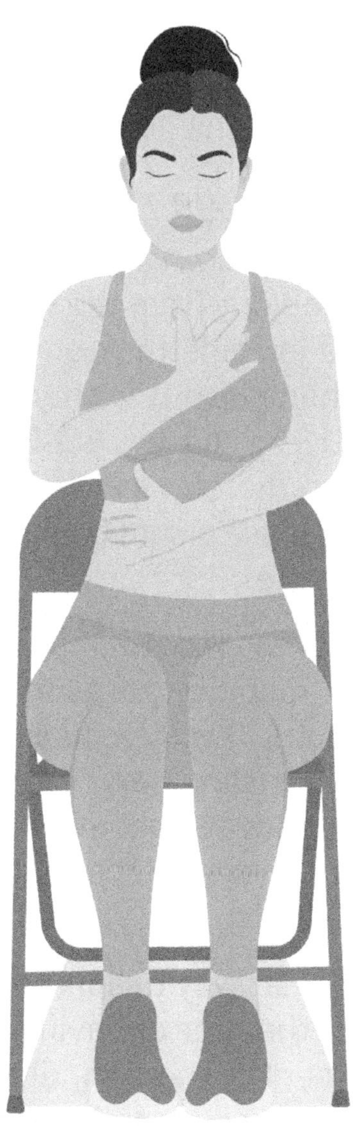

Sit high in your chair with your feet flat on the ground.

Place one hand on your stomach and the other on your chest.

Inhale slowly through the nose, filling the stomach first and then the chest. Slowly exhale through the nose, emptying first the chest and then the stomach.

Repeat this through three breath cycles.

Alternating nostril breathing

This is the second exercise, also called nadi shodhana pranayama.

This exercise helps clear your mind and improve concentration.

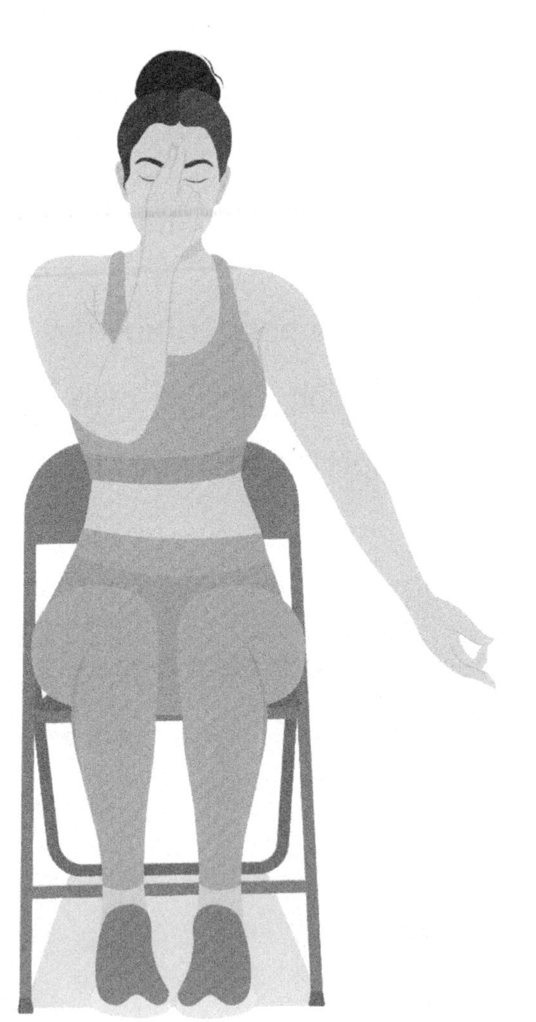

To do this exercise, sit high in your chair with both feet flat on the ground. Placeyour right hand in front of your face and close the right nostril with your thumb.Take a full breath while breathing in leisurely through the left nostril. Then close the left nostril with the ring forefinger and free the right nostril. Gradually breathe out from the right nostril. Breathe in again through the right nostril, then close it with your thumb and delivery the left nostril. Breathe out from theleft nostril. This is a cycle. Repeat for a sum of three to five breath cycles.

Chair yoga is a great way to improve flexibility and mobility, especially among older adults. If you are looking for help with your shoulders, spine, neck, or upperbody in general for more flexibility, then you should try this practice.

Chair yoga is a great way to approach exercise and keep fit without getting stressed. Without the fear of having to achieve results at all costs, without facingthe embarrassment of the gym. Chair yoga serves to rediscover oneself, to become aware, to rediscover and to feel one's body. We know that often those with weight problems tend to forget about themselves, not to look in the mirror.With yoga you must necessarily get back in touch with yourself you must learn tobreathe and feel your breath, feel your body and your mind. Yoga helps you to achieve awareness of yourself, it helps you to accept yourself, and it is preciselyfor this reason that it can bring serious benefits even in weight loss, because weknow that at the base of eating disorders and overweight there is often a bad relationship with the self. This is why losing weight with yoga is possible becauseit guides you to get back in touch with yourself.

Chair yoga is useful because it brings you closer to yoga practices without creating embarrassment, without inducing performance anxiety in a gentle and natural way.

Unlock the Taste of Wellness!

Scan the QR code below to access an exclusive selection of **QUICK AND HEALTHY RECIPES**, perfectly complementing your journey with Chair Yoga.

Enjoy enhancing your wellness journey with flavors that nourish your body and soul.

THANK YOU FOR PURCHASING THIS BOOK, IF YOU ENJOY THIS TITLE, THEN FEEDBACK ON AMAZON WOULD BE GREATLY APPRECIATED.

We want our books to be truly enjoyable for everyone.

Made in the USA
Las Vegas, NV
21 March 2024